A FLICK OF HOPE
Inside Our Reciprocal IVF Story

All Rights Reserved

COPYRIGHT © 2024 Angelita Cusatis

This book may not be reproduced, transmitted, or stored in whole or in part by any means, including graphic, electronic, or mechanical, without the express written consent of the publisher except in the case of brief questions embodied in critical articles and reviews.

This is a work of non-fiction. The events shared are to the best of the author's recollection. Some dialogue and events may be compressed, and some names have been changed to protect the privacy of the people involved.

Paperback ISBN: 979-8-218-35665-1
Hardcover ISBN: 979-8-218-35666-8
Ebook ASIN: B0CTGKY62S

Cover design by Ryan Olson | IG: ryanlucasolson_arts

Additional cover design by Sooraj Mathew

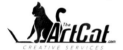

Edited by Hilary Jastram | www.bookmarkpub.com

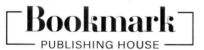

GET IN TOUCH

- Facebook: https://www.facebook.com/angelitacusatisauthor
- Instagram: http://instagram.com/angelitacusatisauthor/
- Email: aflickofhopebook@gmail.com

DEDICATION

To my dear son, Caden Joseph. Follow your heart and your dreams, and find something good in every day. I am so proud of you and will always be grateful that you chose me to be your mommy!

EARLY PRAISE FOR
A FLICK OF HOPE

"Angelita takes the reader on a journey filled with hope, sadness, and, ultimately, joy. She shares her innermost feelings about every part of the infertility process, from selecting a clinic, choosing a sperm donor, undergoing more procedures than she and her wife ever imagined, and the ups and downs of both pregnancy and loss. The joy of their happy ending is that much more profound for what they had to endure to get there. Both she and Dina, her wife, share their personal, heartfelt story with the hope it will inspire anyone who is on their own infertility journey, whether at the beginning, middle, or end. They want anyone reading this book to not feel alone, and they have most assuredly succeeded."

—**Megan Cole**, Marketing Manager—
Fairfax Cryobank

"In Angelita Cusatis's debut memoir, she shares her innermost thoughts as she navigates finding love and building the family she has always wished for. She candidly shares details on the struggles of being in her thirties, looking for love as a same-sex couple, and the trials and tribulations of having a child in her thirties with the help of fertility specialists. Angelita's story is a must-read for any woman who has experienced issues trying to conceive a child, whether in a same-sex or heterosexual *relationship. Her innermost thoughts likely echo those who have shared in the excitement, anticipation, and anxiety of starting their journey to motherhood. With each passing chapter, you feel her emotions, understand her thoughts, and the reasons why she continued to persevere, regardless of the emotional and physical trauma endured. The love shown between her and her partner, Dina, inspires during a time when happy, healthy relationships are hard to come by. This is a love story with an outcome that will leave you awe-inspired."*

—**Anh Kha**, Training Specialist—
Lead Radiation Therapist, New York Proton Center

"A Flick of Hope touches on the thoughts, feelings, hardships, and challenges that so many experience when starting a family. Angelita's story takes you on a journey through all the emotions that couples face—especially those with added challenges—when trying to start a family: IVF, IUI, the successes, the failures, the emotions, family challenges, and pregnancy loss. As someone who has experienced this type of loss, this story covers the highs and lows you go through during the journey of pregnancy. Angelita really dives into the raw emotions that so many out there go through silently; she reminds us that everyone has their struggles, but there is always hope. Her story is a beautifully honest depiction of the road to take when life may not go as planned and how to make the best out of hard situations."

—**Brittani Scott**, Senior Radiation Therapist R.T.(T).—
Maryland Proton Treatment Center

"When I first picked up A Flick of Hope, I wasn't quite sure what to expect. I certainly didn't think I'd pick it up and not be able to put it down until I finished it. The baseline story is about a loving couple's struggle to start a family. The challenges they faced seem, at times, to be too much to take. But they persevered and were rewarded with a beautiful baby boy.

A FLICK OF HOPE
Inside Our Reciprocal IVF Story

Angelita Cusatis

Their story is an inspiration for all couples going through similar circumstances. But it's so much more than that. I found that there are lessons for all of us to learn inside this book. I loved A Flick of Hope!"

—**Jim McAllister**, Commercial Construction Consultant

"A Flick of Hope is a must-read for anyone who dreams of being a parent. The book especially provided inspiration to me, as my husband and I have struggled with infertility and are on our own IVF journey. It truly helped me work through some of my feelings and emotions, and most of all—it offered me hope when I have felt, at times, there was no hope left. While reading, I truly felt like I was on Angelita's journey with her every step of the way. She doesn't hold anything back in this book, which I truly appreciated, as it made me realize just how much someone can handle on their way to parenthood to get that most perfect baby. Angelita shared her feelings of hope, loss, grief, pain, and love, among others. I highly recommend this book, as it will help you feel like you are not alone in your journey—whatever path your journey has taken you on thus far."

—**Lisa Kalodner**, Pharmaceutical Sales Representative— Pfizer, Inc.

"Reading *A Flick of Hope* brought back a rush of emotions as someone who participated in the IVF process with my wife for our only child. Angelita's heartfelt storytelling beautifully captures the vulnerability and hope that come with the journey to motherhood. Her openness about challenges, decisions, and the complexities of relationships resonates deeply with me. Thank you for sharing your journey, vulnerability, and hope."

—**Ron Howard**, Realtor and Author— Greatest Moves Team of RE/MAX Advantage Realty

TABLE OF CONTENTS

Introduction	1
Chapter 1: The Wink	3
Chapter 2: Baby-Making Business	13
Chapter 3: The Perfect Donor	23
Chapter 4: Sixth Time's the Charm	31
Chapter 5: Shadows Fall	41
Chapter 6: The Promise	49
Chapter 7: Hope	57
Chapter 8: The First Transfer	71
Chapter 9: The Line is Bold	81
Chapter 10: Not Beating the Odds	89
Chapter 11: I Can't Tell You How or When	97
Chapter 12: Right Under Our Noses	105
Chapter 13: Caden	119
Acknowledgments	129
About the Author	133

INTRODUCTION

I am a believer that God writes our story at birth.

As much as we want to steal the pen, he has all control, and it is up to us to have the faith.

The experience of writing this book has been incredibly humbling for me. It has been healing in ways I never imagined.

I have learned so much about myself in the process that I will continue to carry into my future.

I am no longer ashamed of some parts.

I am still learning to deal with others.

I learned to honor where I am in life, to allow myself grace when needed, and live in the moments. I have learned to take each day as it comes and not to concern myself too much with the what-ifs.

You don't have to be perfect to inspire others. Sometimes, people are inspired by the way you handle your struggles, heartache, and imperfections.

When my life changed irrevocably, I knew my wife and my family and friends couldn't save me from my pain and that I needed to reach deep and do the work on myself to get back to a healthier place.

Trauma can be crippling if you allow it. It is okay to fall, but it's important to rise again.

Life can throw unforeseen events at us that force us to grow, evolve, and expand our way of thinking about what should be.

Too many times throughout my journey to motherhood, I felt powerless, but that brought with it a sense of humbleness.

When I thought about writing this book and sat down to do so, I did it not only to document my story. I also felt compelled to share it with the ultimate hope of inspiring others on their journey, whether they are at the beginning, middle, or end. The dark days ahead of me turned into my greatest gift in life.

So much shame surrounds infertility, loss, miscarriage, and even stillbirth. I hope my openness, rawness, and vulnerability can help others not feel so alone in theirs.

I want to bring awareness to a topic not spoken about often and provide support and guidance to a relatable audience. No matter your ethnicity, age, or sexual orientation, you are not alone.

I am here.

I want to hold your hand.

I am your advocate, ear, and biggest cheerleader.

I am sending you love, courage, determination, patience, grit, and hope that miracles do happen. But please remember, with a baby or without, you are valuable, you are whole, and you have a life worth living to its fullest.

CHAPTER 1

The Wink

"Love will come. The right person has the key."
—Unknown

When I first saw my wife, Dina, with her stunning hazel eyes and blonde hair, I hoped she wanted a family.

I guess that's why I couldn't wait to talk about it with her. We discussed it even before meeting in person.

I've known since I was a little girl that I wanted to be a mom, but the years were ticking by, and it hadn't happened. After a turn on the relationship merry-go-round, I was determined to do things differently. I was just missing one thing. I needed to meet the right girl first.

Now, I thank God having kids didn't happen before I met my person. If you're reading this and feeling like you will never find your other half, hang in there because sometimes, it takes a minute.

Dina and I were on the same page right away. The closer we got, the more we knew it was meant to be.

When I say Dina and I were on a mission to be with each other, I am not exaggerating. She moved in with me seven months after we started dating.

The following year, she proposed to me. I knew it was coming. I just didn't know *what* was coming and when.

It was during our second trip together out of the country. We were in Cancun, Mexico, for the week. Dina had bought the ring and planned to ask me during this trip.

It was one of our last evenings, during the most romantic sunset on our suite's balcony. She got down on one knee (I am a sucker for the old-fashioned ways) and asked me in the sweetest way.

She was so nervous yet so confident at the same time. I was swooning at the thought of my dream girl walking down the aisle to meet me, ready to spend the rest of our lives together. I could picture the wedding and how gorgeous she would look and our amazing life together. I was over-the-moon giddy.

Is this really happening?

But I was ready for it all with her! The good, the bad, the ugly, the beautiful moments. Everything that comes when you commit yourself to someone and share a life with them.

Dina and I met on match.com. I was casually dating, and Dina had been in and out of relationships for some time. She winked at me, and that's all it took.

Normally, I would engage in a little small talk, like "Hi, how are you?" But it was just a wink at first sight, so I figured our communication would be kind of shallow.

There might be a mutual attraction, but I didn't expect anything. Little did I know on the other end of the chat was my dream girl.

Physically, she was absolutely my type. But would I be hers? I had to wonder: *Does she even have a type?* It was surprising how fast Dina got in my head.

Honestly, I didn't read what she had to say on her profile bio. I didn't even know where she lived. I just assumed she lived somewhere local because I hadn't put my radius out that far. By then, I'd had quite a few long-distance relationships in my life—probably intentionally. But for the first time, I didn't want to do that anymore. The drive and time invested going back and forth driving hundreds of miles were exhausting. It was time to change it up.

I winked back, then Dina messaged, and I finally read her profile. *Wow, she sounds pretty interesting. Not only is she very attractive, but I like what she has to say.* My thoughts of her intensified.

Then we started chatting on the phone. Our friends laugh now when we talk about those early days. Our conversation was heavy. I was not in the mood to play around since I'd just come out of a bad breakup.

It's ironic I write that because when I signed up for match.com, I wanted casual, but something deep inside me wanted more—seeing Dina's photo forced me to realize that. Dina and I spent hours on the phone every day getting to know each other outside of the physical parts of a relationship. We would stay up until midnight every night.

We have so many likes in common, yet we are so opposite personality-wise. I am your Type A alpha, and she is a perfect blend of all personality types. I am the lay-your-shoes-next-to-each-other person, and she has the kick-your-shoes-off-and-wherever-they-land-I'll-get-to-them-later mindset. It's cute. Although, on some occasions, it's not so much when I end up tripping over them. Dina is the protector and nurturer. She is altruistic. I am the planner, get-er-done, handle-things-like-a-boss kind of girl. We are both extremely independent and opinionated yet emotional and empathetic. The whole time I was talking to her, I felt she was my match and thought, *this girl is a genuine soul.* I quickly realized *she is a woman of her word.* Before long, she became my calm, my rationale.

My ex and I really started talking about having kids after we were engaged. She proposed to me about three years into dating. Then, it all fell apart. I'd ask her, "When are we going to get married? My biological clock is ticking. I'm 32, and you're 34."

You obviously know how that ended. Long story short, she led me on all that time, telling me she wanted a family and kids, too. But it wasn't true. I was not about to go through that again and showed all my cards to Dina. *You're in, or you're out.*

It paid off in the beginning, and it's paying off now. There's something to be said about being direct. Dina and I firmly believe communication really is the key to a healthy relationship. As we got deeper and deeper into it, we nurtured a phenomenal relationship. It was everything I had ever wanted. We were so much in love; I fell hard and quick. Our families loved each other, too. My head was spinning with all the goodness. It was so perfect.

Every date and day were so much fun. We went out to dinner, got coffee, and enjoyed long walks and chatting away as we got to know more of each other.

We traveled a lot for fun, and when Dina ran a few races in other cities—I went with her for support. We went to concerts and spent a lot of time with each other's families and friends. Before we made the long drive back home from seeing each other every weekend, we made sure to have early Sunday dinners with each other's families.

It all went against the non-committal-attitude I intended to keep after my breakup. There were three things I wasn't going to budge on, which had everything to do with why I didn't want to date long-distance. Dina, living three-and-a-half hours away in Pennsylvania, broke one of those rules. I didn't know how that would work or if it would work. I did know I was not moving because my family is here. My job is here, and I have spent many years building my career.

That's why when we first started talking, I said, "Please, don't waste my time." I knew what I wanted and didn't want. And even though I thought I would play around and not get serious, when I met Dina, all the pieces clicked into place. It was either get serious or get out. Just when I thought I knew what I wanted, it turned out I didn't have a clue what I was looking for.

It was like stepping out onto a branch and hoping it held my weight. I didn't want to get hurt, but I didn't want to give up my dreams. So, I would risk flying even if I fell on my face.

My relationship had ended a little over a year before, and it was devastating. I'd been strung along for so long that I'd actually told my ex, "It's okay if you don't want the same things I do. I can be happy. We can still be content together."

When she looked at me, I knew what was coming. "I love you more than you know, but I can't be in a relationship with you where you have to give up having kids." It made sense, and I respect her for her honesty, but it destroyed me at the time. The saying, "Don't give up your dreams for someone else's sake," resonates hard with me to this day. But there I was, trying again and so afraid of getting hurt. That's why I laid it on the line with Dina. I just kept thinking *you want this, but you don't want to get hurt.* All I could do was walk forward, and thankfully, Dina walked with me.

Now, when we reflect on those days, Dina admits it was intense, although she wanted the same things. But at the time, it was all I knew to do—protect my heart while trying to keep the spark going with her.

The first time we were to meet was on a Saturday. Before our date, Dina messaged me and said, "I don't know if this is a good idea with the distance, and I'm really busy with my job and training."

I knew she had a ton going on. In addition to her full-time work, she was a personal trainer and a Zumba and spin instructor on the side. She also comes from a very big family, which took up her time. Dina is very family-oriented. It's one of the qualities I absolutely adore about her. But at that moment, I wasn't crazy about her canceling on me—even though she had good reasons. I was crushed and annoyed.

We were going to meet at a halfway point at a casino in Hershey, Pennsylvania, where her sister lives. I thought she'd really want to go because she loves to gamble. Maybe I was baiting the hook, thinking if I played my cards right, I would score another date.

After she canceled, I was pretty riled up about it and talked to one of my best friends, Crystal, as we nursed drinks at a bar. I told her, "Who does this girl think she is? I kept replaying Dina's words as I tried to read more into what she'd said: "I'm not quite sure if I should take you seriously, and I want to believe you. But at the same time, why are you single? You're very attractive. You live in Baltimore City. I would imagine there are many lesbians in Baltimore."

Keeping in mind that Dina was the one who winked first at me and that she knew how far away I lived, I had to wonder, *is Dina trying to protect her heart as well?*

I rolled my eyes as we spoke on the phone and said, "Sure there is—just like any other big city. But that doesn't necessarily mean I want to date anyone here. The community isn't as big as you would think, and everyone kind of hooks up with each other, or they've dated each other. I don't want to date someone knowing they've already slept with five people in the same room."

At that moment, as those words were coming out of my mouth, I realized one of the reasons I'd always started long-distance relationships.

The less I know about the past, the better.

"Well, I think you might be a player, and I don't know if I should take you seriously or if you're sincere." *Ouch.*

Then she canceled. Bottom line, I couldn't figure her out. And I couldn't forget that she had canceled what was to be our first date. That was the first time in my life that had ever happened. My ego was a bit bruised.

Flash forward to my friend Crystal and me drowning our sorrows together. We were both in the same headspace. She wanted to set her ex-boyfriend's stuff on fire, and I was peeved over being dumped before we even got going.

Shots flew as we dissected our personal situations.

As I tried to wrap my head around what had happened with Dina, I looked at Crystal and said, "Why would she do this? What's wrong with me? Am I not pretty? I mean, what is it?" Again, she had winked at and messaged me first.

Crystal peered at me like I was crazy. "Stop it. You're gorgeous. You know that? If I was a lesbian, I'd date you in a heartbeat."

I gave her a small smile and swirled my shot glass. "Do I look like a player? Do my pictures make me seem that way? Is it because I live in Baltimore City? Was it something I said or didn't say? Is it because I really didn't write much in my profile bio? I mean, my motto is, 'If you want to know more, just ask.'"

I wouldn't stop pestering Crystal, and I have to thank her for taking the next step. As I got up to go to the bathroom, she took my phone and texted Dina: "You don't know what you're missing. Ang is one of a kind. She is really sincere and has a heart of gold. I wish you would reconsider."

Dina messaged back, "I appreciate everything you're saying, and I'm sure she is great. I'm just not quite sure about the distance and my schedule and everything I have going on in my life, if it would even be the most appropriate time, but who knows what the future holds?"

When I came back, Crystal had this weird expression on her face. "So, I did a thing." She smiled in that way that I knew meant she was asking for forgiveness.

I sat down slowly. "What did you do?" And she showed me my phone. My heart sank and lightened at the same time. *Who knows what the future holds?*

Crystal stood up and grabbed my hand. "You know what? That girl doesn't deserve you. Let's get on the dance floor." You'll find someone else," Crystal said confidently.

Let me just point out that we were at a straight bar. I followed her out to the floor, but I wasn't in the mood.

Then, when I got home, totally out of character for me, I messaged Dina. I'm not normally the pursuer, but I was breaking the rules for her.

She called me back and opened the conversation with, "What is wrong with you, calling me at 3:00 a.m.? I have to go in early to treat a patient." Dina is Italian, and I heard that side come out for the first time.

I said, "I might be a little drunk. Not gonna lie."

"I don't care if you're drunk, but why are you so cute?"

I didn't know what to say to that. *She thinks I'm cute! Is being the pursuer attractive?* My pounding heart told me I liked that.

Dina said, "I'm really sorry. And just so you know, I stayed in and made tacos tonight and watched *The Intern*. I did not go out like you did."

That got me. My anger flared for a second. *How is she talking to me like this when she is the one who canceled on me?*

"Here we go. You think I'm a player because I went out looking for something, but *you* canceled on me. If I were doing something, I would be somewhere else. Or someone would be with me. And I clearly wouldn't be texting you at 3:00 a.m. from home."

She saw my point.

Thankfully, the conversation took a nicer turn.

That following morning, just a couple of hours later, she messaged me a picture of herself.

As I stared at it, I thought, *I'm back in*.

She was, too, even though our plans to meet the second time fell through—but that's a story for another time. Weirdly, we did not meet in person for quite a while.

Once we were all in, our calls and texts got so intense it was inevitable we would meet.

We were never really apart again after meeting for the first time and saw each other every single weekend after that. We would alternate weekends at each other's places and head back home Sunday afternoon, so we could get to work on Monday. That equated to a seven-hour drive in under 48 hours. We did this every weekend for seven months, except for two weekends—Mother's Day and the weekend Dina packed up and moved to Baltimore.

That's right, Dina moved here—even though she'd had an amazing job for 14-plus years with equally amazing hours. Dina gave up a lot to come here and be with me.

When we read our vows, I promised to make sure that every day she wouldn't feel any regrets. I knew what she had sacrificed, picking up her life and moving it here, to a big city to live in an environment she had never been in before. It was especially significant at her age. She was 38, and it was a struggle for a bit to get settled in and find her bearings, but then it all worked out.

She is now the chief therapist at the same cancer center she started with after moving here seven years ago. To see this opportunity for her warms my heart. It was not all in vain; she's excelling in her career and married, and after trekking an arduous road in the fertility world, she has a beautiful son. Oh yeah, and she has me.

Dina and I were destined to be together, and if you keep reading, you will find out about the most incredible gift we have given each other. I hope you do.

CHAPTER 2

Baby-Making Business

> *"Making the decision to have a child is momentous.
> It is to decide forever to have your heart go walking
> around outside your body."*
> —Elizabeth Stone

As our relationship grew, the plan was for me to carry our child. We never considered any other way at the start. Dina had no desire to carry, and having a biological kid didn't matter to her. That worked out for me since all I wanted to do was carry. I'd dreamed about it since I understood what getting pregnant meant. In those dreams, I saw myself as the mother of baby girls. But I needed more.

Growing up, I always envisioned and wanted to have three kids. The start of our family would be a perfect baby—I could see it in my mind. I was so determined to have children that before I met Dina, I was seriously thinking about taking the steps to have a family of my own without a partner.

We thought my carrying would be the perfect arrangement. In my heart, I'd finally met the girl of my dreams. Dina was everything

I was looking for. We had insane chemistry, *and* she wanted kids? I finally felt understood and like I had a real shot at this mom thing.

The plan was to get down to baby-making business a couple of months after we got married.

However you decide to get pregnant, we all know it can take time, and as we were about to learn, it can also take you on quite a journey.

If we had both been younger, we would have enjoyed being married and traveling more, but the clock was ticking the second we said our vows in August 2018, and we knew it.

That next January, after our wedding, we were all ready. New year, new us, new baby. The timing seemed perfect. All my childhood dreams were about to come true.

After researching which fertility clinic to use, we went with Shady Grove Fertility and made an appointment. It's well-renowned and one of the best. Kind of an important criterion when you are about to grow a baby.

Our doctor was matter-of-fact, intelligent, scientific, and even endearing, which we weren't expecting. As a same-sex couple, we weren't sure how we would be treated—even though it's the 21st century (come on!), but he was absolutely lovely, and we felt no different than any other couple about to embark on one of their biggest milestones.

The first appointment was like an interview. We drilled him on everything we wanted to know. And this is a critical point—don't put all your eggs in one basket—literally. Make sure you have a second and even a third clinic picked out if your first choice doesn't work out. Our second choice was Johns Hopkins Fertility Center—a solid alternative.

But there would be no second choice. Shady Grove was it. From the minute we walked in, we hit it off with the doctor. He was just as excited for us! He went over everything, which was extremely overwhelming, but we were both somewhat prepared. Having friends making their families the new-fashioned way will rub off on you. And Dina and I were very curious about their experiences so we could try to anticipate our own.

When you start the long and involved process of figuring out how to have a baby using a fertility clinic, it takes a lot of research and is exhausting emotionally and financially. It doesn't matter if you're a same-sex or heterosexual couple. It's not a service that's easy to afford unless you have amazing insurance. Luckily, that was the case for us. I had coverage through my work, and Dina and I were both covered through the hospital where she worked. With dual insurance, we paid $950 in monthly premiums for three years. We still had to pay out of pocket for co-pays and all the additional fees insurance didn't cover, which amounted to about $25,000.

Do yourself a huge favor if you are ready to take this step. Although the fertility clinic's financial coordinator will help you through the insurance aspect, you also need to explore all your options and coverages separately. Navigating through insurance can be arduous. Using keywords and accurate codes will make all the difference in the information you receive from your insurance providers.

That was the case for us, but it's different for everyone. Some of my friends have spent $50,000 plus out-of-pocket for one child because they didn't have good insurance. Just know I understand if you're beginning this journey, it can be discouraging.

That was one consideration we had to come to terms with. Another was who would be our donor.

From the day we stepped foot into the clinic, we tossed around ideas of what we would want our donor to look like and the characteristics we wanted him to have.

We always thought we'd select somebody as close as possible to Dina because this would be my biological baby, so I knew I'd be represented—but we wanted a blend of us.

Since Dina is the All-American girl, we needed a donor who resembled a tall blonde man with hazel eyes. We figured he would be extremely athletic, too. Searching for a donor and writing down your criteria is your chance to build a perfect guy. There are thousands of donors out there to choose from, so we had a lot of work ahead of us.

Our heterosexual friends laughed and were intrigued at the whole process, saying, "I didn't get to pick my husband's traits. He's not the hottest guy. *Don't tell him that!*"

It wasn't just his physical attributes we had to get right. This is the deepest dive into a person you've ever taken. We're talking about their physical and mental health history; you need to know if they've had any diseases, all about their genetics, and so forth.

And we knew there was no one perfect guy. But between August and January, our life was about constructing a flawless man to help us achieve our dream. Ironic as a lesbian couple and good for a chuckle.

I couldn't wait to get started because I'd transformed into young teenage me with the butterflies thinking about having kids and carrying. I always pictured myself as a girl mom, but what they say is true. You don't know what you want. The Universe, however, knows what you need.

I wanted to feel the kicks and the growth, too, and I was so anxious to wear the cute little pregnancy clothes, but the bigger picture for me was the attachment—knowing that I would carry this precious child and we would be one being for nine months.

My wanting to carry made for a very easy conversation to have. There was no discussion, but more like a plan unfolding, and while we thought everything would go off without a hitch—barring the usual pregnancy surprises—like morning sickness and fatigue—we were in for a shock.

Since our appointment was in January, I did the math, figuring we would get pregnant by April or May. That's the classic planner side of me. Looking back. I almost feel conceited and a little foolish. When you're knocking on 40, it's not as easy to get pregnant. But then again, I was basing my assessment on heterosexual females and couples. We were getting a direct drop-off; our sperm would be inserted precisely where it needed to go. I thought *this has to be quicker. These people know what they're doing. They're just going to inseminate me and send me on my way, and I'm gonna get pregnant—like that day!*

I was kinda right. But first, there was the screw-up with my insurance company. Unless I had proof of coverage, they wouldn't see us. The insurance company had not sent over the required paperwork, so we were SOL when we arrived for the January appointment. I burst into tears. I had built up so much hope and expectation for this day—*only to be sent home?*

As I struggled to compose myself, Dina grabbed my hand in that way she has and, softly yet firmly, said, "Look at it this way. What if this is the only time we ever walk out of this fertility clinic crying?"

Wham! She has this way of slamming home the truth.

I sniffed a little and sucked up my tears. "Wow, that does make me feel better." Then I managed a smile and said with a hitch in my voice, "I'm still really angry, but I'm also okay."

Her remark gave me hope. My friends have gone through this process, and time and time again, they've walked out of the clinic with bad news. They've been broken and discouraged. That was not us. It was an insurance hang-up, and *we would* get it figured out.

My control freak personality emerged right on cue. *I pledged to myself: This is the only time we'll have a paperwork screw-up.*

Three weeks later, Dina and I made another appointment, and this time, I had a copy of my insurance in hand. If they told me they didn't have it at the clinic, I could give it to them. Check-in was smooth and easy. We took our seats in the waiting room.

So many women surrounded us. We could see sadness in some faces, hope in others, anticipation, despair, and so on. As you might expect, this is a very emotional journey.

As we sat there, Dina and I whispered about each of these women and wondered what had brought them here. Was that single woman who looked engrossed in a women's health magazine dealing with aging eggs? What about that woman over there, curled up in the chair playing on her phone—was it her husband's sperm motility? We wondered if another woman tapping her feet was a single mother who hadn't found her partner. Had she decided it was time to go it alone—was she retrieving frozen eggs to do it? Maybe the put-together woman with the shiny blonde hair across from us was a lesbian and taking that first step like we were?

It was reassuring to see that we weren't alone in our fertility journey. But I was curious if we would have an easier time than a heterosexual couple—who had all the right equipment that wasn't working.

That endearing doctor Dina and I had researched and chosen in Columbia, Maryland, the location nearest our house and my office, was an excellent fit for us. We were now preparing to see him again—this time, to get the baby-making ball rolling.

Once inside his office, the doctor immediately shook our hands and pulled out chairs for Dina and me. He was such a gentleman in his button-up yellow shirt and khaki slacks. I'm a terrible judge of ages, but I guessed him to be in his fifties.

He sat down behind his desk, smiled warmly, and said, "Tell me about yourselves."

Dina and I dove right in and gave him the basics about our life together, and then we got more personal, talking about our ages and health, why we wanted a kid, and so on. I shared that I have MS (multiple sclerosis), and I wasn't sure if that was a factor in sustaining a healthy pregnancy or not. It didn't end up being one—if you are worried about that. Pro tip: Sometimes, what we worry about doesn't matter at all.

I couldn't believe it, but the doctor actually said, "I have numerous patients that have gotten pregnant multiple times with MS, and they've done wonderfully. I don't have any concerns about you. Your case seems very mild, and you're not having symptoms now. Cognitively, everything checks out, and unless something dramatically changes, there's no reason why you wouldn't be able to carry." I smiled at that. I couldn't help it. Okay, maybe I bounced in my chair a little. You would, too, if you were on the cusp of your dreams.

I should mention that prior to seeing this doctor, I was cleared by my primary care doctor. The fertility clinic wants to make sure all your doctors are on board, and all the boxes are checked. My OBGYN also cleared me. Everyone was in agreement: I could get knocked up. The good news: MS has nothing to do with carrying. The only thing you might have to worry about with MS comes after you give birth. The tougher news: Some people can slip into a flare because hormones drastically change and are all over the place. I didn't care. I would deal with that if and when it happened.

With the MS question out of the way, the doctor was off and running, citing statistics and our chance of success based on our ages and health, how long the process usually takes, any complications that might arise, pricing, insurance, and everything else you can imagine might happen at a fertility appointment. It's a mix of sharing your hopes and dreams with your physical potential and science.

We let him talk a lot because that was why we were there, to interview him. As much as he wanted to know everything about us, we wanted to know everything about him. And the connection with this doctor was important. If we weren't feeling it, it was still early enough in the game to find another doctor. It's a little like a job interview. You want to find the best person to help you through a project to get the best results possible. This man was going to be our teammate—but more realistically, he would be our team lead.

He next told us that Shady Grove required all couples to go through counseling because it's an emotional process. It helps to provide resources and support to reduce the stress this process can bring with it. It becomes part of your care team. Whoever is carrying is also pumping up their body full of hormones, and the preparation to get pregnant goes on for what feels like forever. Let me put it this way: You feel like you're fat . . . with eggs.

I was *almost* offended when the doctor told us we would have to go to counseling, and for a split second, I thought we were being targeted as a same-sex couple. Then I told myself: *Calm down*. And as politely as I could, I asked, "Is this a requirement?" as Dina gave me the side-eye.

The doctor just smiled at me like he knew what I meant. "Absolutely. I don't want anyone to come in here and take it lightly like it's just going to happen overnight. We want to make sure that our patients are on the same page. We want everyone to be well-prepared and informed to the best of their ability.

"And," he went on, "there's a fee associated with the counseling. It's not covered by insurance." *Of course, it's not.*

We talked a little more, and I felt good about him helping to bring our baby into the world.

No matter that this doctor was wonderful, warm, and thorough, we left his office overwhelmed, gripping the folder with all the information we needed to know. I was happy to take it home, where I could stay up all night and soak it all in. I had waited this long to feel so over my head, and I was determined to savor every moment of it.

I supposed after reading through the immense pile of information that night, I could start tackling the items on the checklist the next day. A lot of them were geared toward me since I was the one who would be going through the process. Dina's part was to provide the emotional support needed and navigate the insurance company if she had to step in.

After reading everything over and feeling good about the next steps, it was time to sign a contract and set up our second appointment with the clinic. I was ready and just wanted time to move a little faster. Still, it was surreal to think: *I am getting pregnant in a few short months.*

Our next appointment was set for February. It was extremely hard to wait and not drive to the clinic and demand they get going. I half-wanted to ask whoever was in charge, "If I pay an extra fee, will you put me on a priority list?"

Back then, I was such a planner, and mentally, our journey was all worked out in my head. People I've known for decades have since said, "You're funny how you plan out your life—especially when it came to this."

But life and biology do not like to be told what to do. Boy, did I learn that the hard way.

Despite what you are about to read, and even though we rode the roller coaster to get Caden here, I know I am very blessed. Suffering doesn't take away a blessing. Sometimes, it takes the biggest losses to realize that. And although life doesn't always work out as planned, sometimes it works out even better.

CHAPTER 3

The Perfect Donor

"A vial of sperm is in the comparatively reasonable range of $700—and finding the donor you like is not unlike shopping online at J. Crew."
—Unknown (Correction, that's $950 now!)

At least we had something to do between the first appointment and the next one. That time was hot and heavy designing our ideal donor. We threw ourselves into this job—knowing it was one of the most important tasks we would ever do.

Shady Grove recommended three different sperm donation banks to choose from—one in Seattle and another in California, but we were fortunate enough to note another one about an hour away from our house in Fairfax, Virginia—Fairfax Cryobank (with over 35 years of experience helping clients worldwide achieve their family-building dreams) and yes, I know, some people don't have that luxury. I hoped it would have everything we needed. Even if it didn't, the location wouldn't matter. Still, I crossed my fingers because I was digging all this convenience.

Understand the fertility clinic only does the procedures but doesn't offer the eggs or sperm. You're on your own when it comes to getting what you need.

Well, we wanted the best of the best, so we signed up for all three of these places. We paid the monthly membership fee three times. We were not about to put a price on our baby. A quick search of the Fairfax bank gave me limited information, but I couldn't see too much until I paid the fee. By this time, I didn't care about costs, and that was only the tip of it. We had hundreds of donors' information to wade through.

When you sign up with the sperm bank, you will feel like you're flying blind. We had no assistance in the sign-up and had to navigate everything we wanted to do and see. For example, Fairfax Cryobank ranges from $100-150 for basic or full access with a la carte options (yes, you read that right) for 90 days. Which seems reasonable when you consider you're buying a huge part of the essence of human life. I estimated we would need each service for at least 90 days.

Finding our donor would be a long process. Our friends who had already been through this told us, "Have fun with it. This doesn't have to be a super serious process. It's a big deal, yes, but take the edge out of it. Trust the process and each other. Have a glass of wine when you do it." So that's what Dina and I did.

We knew we didn't have to pick someone overnight. The doctor had reiterated that it would be quite a few months before we could get into the physical aspect of it. Between the testing and health workup, the insurance paperwork, and selecting the donor, we had time. Having this big window was not easy for me. In anything else in life, I am the epitome of patience. Not with this.

I had hung tight for decades just to hurry up and wait.

When picking a donor, you start with a broad sampling and narrow it down. Before you sift through any of the ID profiles, make sure you've written down your deal-breakers and what's super important to you. Height, hair color, eye color, education, and religion might be important, for instance. Once we narrowed down our handful of guys, we hit it hard and went through each one with a fine-tooth comb. We were paying good money for this privilege, so we didn't waste a moment or chance to engage with it deeply.

Starting with the broad search, as you might imagine, is a little shallow, but let's be honest, it's how everyone goes about their life when they want to connect with another person. You see what they have to offer on the outside.

As Dina and I looked through the donors' baby pictures, we drank our wine and would grin at each other and say, "Oh my goodness, what a cutie!" "Isn't he adorable?" "I just want to eat him up!"

We kept scrolling as the pictures gave way to aging kids. Then, they turned into teenagers in that awkward stage. Not quite as adorable, but we were still open to what we were seeing because, *hey, who didn't have that phase?* You don't want to see a picture of me in middle school!

Finally, you get to see the donors' adult pictures, which means you come face-to-face with your judgments. Your most loving motivation is that you want to have a baby, but you have to confront your judgment of how you want your baby to look, and you don't *really* want to go down that road—because, of course, you want a healthy baby—but you're human, so you do.

Some donors are anonymous. You can't find out any information about them because the sperm bank has interviewed them and taken measures to protect them. The clinics are not just taking any random guy off the street who comes in and wants to make money, either.

I read that sperm banks are often clustered around universities where many intelligent and virile young men live. And those clinics are thorough!

Donors complete a rigorous screening process. In fact, Fairfax Cryobank states only one in 200 applicants make it through the process to become a donor, including a physical exam, an in-person interview to review family medical history, and blood, semen, genetic, and infectious disease testing. It is not a quick process for the donors by any means.

We have about 50 pages worth of our donor's information going all the way back to his great-grandparents, including their ages, hair color, eye color, what they did for a living, if they've had Alzheimer's, and any and everything else. The only thing we do not have on this gentleman is his name and address.

To make it even more complicated, we chose what's called an ID Option Donor—I'll explain more below. This was very important to Dina and me when selecting a donor. It means you can see pictures of your donor from when they were a baby up until adulthood.

We have, in total, eleven pictures of our donor as he's growing. We don't have baby pictures; for some reason, he didn't submit any of those. But we can see what he looks like starting at two years old. He's adorable, and we think he's the most handsome guy in the world.

There are varying packages that allow you to see the maximum amount of information allowed, and others are more conservative. What you pick is up to you. Remember that a la carte option I spoke about earlier?

An ID Option Donor signs a contract agreeing that the sperm bank can release their identity—name, DOB, address, and contact information—to the donor-conceived child once that child reaches the age of 18. Then, they can reach out to the sperm bank for information about the donor. If the donor is open to one form of contact, that can happen, too. These donors are required to update their personal information yearly with the sperm bank, as well.

Fun fact: Today, about 45% of donors are ID Option for personal or medical reasons. Before 2005, all donors were anonymous. [1]

At some point, our child will question, "Who is my dad? We want to be ready. First, we don't call him dad—that's another conversation—he is our sperm donor. He has no involvement in raising Caden. We will tell him, "Mommies needed help to start our family and have you. We sought his help. This sweet man helped bring you into this world, and we will be forever grateful to him because we have you." We want to be upfront with Caden about his background.

I can imagine another conversation with an older Caden. "This guy has some cool attributes. He was a wrestler from the ages of five through college, was on the Dean's List, and was a wrestling referee at the time of his donation. He is a project manager. That's very similar to what your mommy does. He also loves all sports, especially wrestling, football, hockey, and baseball. And he loves horses and racing. He spent summers on his family's farm and at his aunt's and uncle's veterinary clinic, working and taking care of animals. The sperm bank described him as a little reserved at first but adventurous and strong-willed, with a confident demeanor. We know he also has a warm, charming personality with an enchanting smile. He loves to cook and be at the lake. His favorite music genre is classic rock, and his favorite song is 'Beast of Burden' by the Rolling Stones. You know Mama Dina loves classic rock, too."

---

1 "What Is an ID Donor?: Fairfax Cryobank." Fairfax Cryobank - Find a Sperm Donor, August 3, 2021. https://fairfaxcryobank.com/blog/uncategorized/what-is-an-id-donor.

We can show him pictures to close some of the loops in his mind. He has a right to be informed about this person who helped give him life. The sperm bank did not have a celebrity look-a-like for him, but one of our friends said he resembles Tom Brady. Tom Brady, who? Just playing!!

Dina and I feel very strongly about having open communication, which extends to our child. This is a key strength in any relationship, and we are committed to never hiding anything from Caden . . . even if that means navigating awkward waters and sometimes not having the answers.

It took a good month to get our donors down to two men. It helped that there weren't as many to choose from as we had thought once we narrowed them down.

The two guys came down to our donor in Virginia and another man in California. They both resembled Dina, but we went with our donor because he looked so wholesome.

His spending a lot of time on a farm as a kid just screams All-American good guy. We love that he loves animals, too.

The other guy was good-looking and reminded us of a tan and blonde Cali surfer dude. There was legit, a picture of him on a surfboard. Coming from a lesbian, California dude was fine, but he was missing the wholesome piece. And we were torn in trying to plan the height of our child. If we had a girl, we didn't want her to be too tall. If we had a boy, we wanted him to be tall. California dude was over six feet, and our donor is 5'10", so that was one of the deciding factors.

The night we narrowed the donor list to those two was the night we picked our donor. It was that fast because we loved him and almost fell *in* love with him. Besides, he *really could be* Dina's brother based on his facial features alone: the same nose, cheeks, and chin. It was crazy.

We paid an additional fee to do what's called FaceMatch.[2] We loaded Dina's photo into the program, and it used a technology algorithm to find a sperm donor lookalike. These days, is there anything not available out there at a cost?

We loved our donor even more when we listened to his voice. The sperm bank gives you a 30-minute recorded audio interview (if you pay for it), and you can listen to how your potential donor answers questions. This guy sounded wise beyond his years and extremely educated.

When he was asked, "Why did you decide to donate sperm?" we swooned over his reply. He said something along the lines of: " My first exposure to learning about becoming a donor was during a biomedical ethics class in college where we learned about human experimentation, fetal research, and reproductive technologies. My close female friend needed help starting her family, and so did my roommate's brother and his wife. They required the egg and the sperm. That inspired me, and I wished I could have helped my friend, but that would have been a very weird, awkward situation. Then I thought if I could be the source of helping other families out there, I would love to do so."

That was it for us. He was in.

---

2   "Fairfax FaceMatch®." Fairfax Cryobank - Find a Sperm Donor, August 12, 2021. https://fairfaxcryobank.com/fairfax-facematch.

CHAPTER 4

Sixth Time's the Charm

"You may have to fight a battle more than once to win it."
—Margaret Thatcher

It was time for the next steps: Purchasing vials of sperm and letting the fertility clinic know we'd chosen our donor.

Pending all my test results that I was fit to carry, I would start the IUI (intrauterine insemination) process. The IUI and IVF (in-vitro fertilization) processes are different from each other in that the semen is placed in the uterus in IUI, and with IVF, the eggs are retrieved from the woman's ovaries, fertilized with the sperm in a dish inside the laboratory, and watched to ensure they grow to a blastocyst stage. Then they're placed into the uterus, where, hopefully, they will grow into embryos.

My testing came back perfectly. Our doctor said, "Angelita, I see absolutely no reason why we could not get you pregnant. Statistically, given your age of 37, I think it's going to take around five to six IUI tries." That was all I needed to hear.

In five or six rounds, I will be pregnant! echoed in my head.

Our doctor also didn't think IVF would be necessary, which was great news, as that procedure is much more invasive.

The plan was to let Shady Grove put the very expensive sperm into a catheter and inseminate my uterus. It's basically a fancy upgrade of the turkey baster at-home process, which surprisingly works for some couples. Sounds easy enough, right? Well, there is a lot more to it than that.

After that, I would just hope and pray that the millions of little spermies swimming in there would attach to the one egg I released when I ovulated. Remember that movie *Look Who's Talking* with John Travolta and Kirstie Alley? All I saw and wanted was the opening credit scene!

Even though it might seem like the odds were stacked in our favor—at literally millions to one, the success rates for IUI are low. That's because the sperm must be frozen, shipped, thawed, and inserted. After it's frozen then thawed, it only lives for about 24 hours inside the uterus. On the flip side, fresh sperm live for as long as five days.

When the nurse told us to order the sperm, I was thrown into confusion. This is not like ordering socks off Amazon. For all the tries you're going to do—and you don't know how many that will be until one of the implantations sticks—the clinic wants to ensure you will have enough. Whatever you order predicates how many tries you get. The doc had said he thought try five or six would be the magic number, so I ordered seven to be on the safe side and felt confident we would be successful quickly.

I thought I had all sorts of positive factors on my side: I'd never been on birth control—I don't know, maybe I thought my uterus was extra chaste? More importantly, my eggs looked healthy, and in late 30-something women, that is not always the case. Egg count and health decline rapidly after the age of 35. In addition, sperm loses motility as men age, which is why those banks scout college guys!

When it came down to ordering, another dilemma hit me. Our donor had seven vials left. It was more than we needed, but I didn't want to be stuck. What if the sixth one didn't take, and I hadn't gotten enough, and then I went back to grab it, and it was gone? What if I got pregnant earlier than expected, but we still needed more to have a second kid? It was one extra vial, and it seemed silly not to take it, so we bought it, too, for a whopping total of $6,650. Besides, believe it or not, you can sell back any unused vials for 50% of what you paid. Each vial is approximately $950, so it adds up. Unfortunately, there was no BOGO.

In retrospect, we could have saved ourselves a lot of money and heartache if we had gone straight to IVF.

In IUI, you get one try a month when you're ovulating, and you're only releasing one egg, but you need an entire vial of sperm. With IVF and egg retrieval, you again need one vial of sperm, but you will likely have eggs—plural. This first procedure was truly a shot in the dark.

Even after we tried to place the sperm order, we weren't done jumping through hoops—and I am telling you, if you want to play this game, you better be great at hoop jumping!

That's right, we *tried* to place the order, but our guy had a waitlist! I didn't even know there was such a thing. We were told if more vials were available, they would let us know. So, our donor's dream of making families a reality for hurting couples has come true. He must have quite a few babies out there. Caden is one.

This whole process of testing and waiting and researching and thinking you have it figured out, but you don't, was really wearing on me—on both of us. I was trying to figure out: *How do I get to be number one on the waitlist? Is there an extra fee I can pay? Because I'm getting pregnant, dammit, and I want that sperm.* By then, I wasn't even settling for surfer dude.

Once the sperm was available again, we upped our order from seven to nine—because you never know. That was the motto of this journey.

Of course, we were crazy. And we hadn't even started the process yet!

We had to buy the sperm, pay to ship it, and fork out $45 for the fertility clinic to store it until it was used. All the costs add up, and it's hard to estimate them when they pop up all over the place. Not to mention, figuring out what costs to include is all up to you. You are in charge of wrangling this whole thing. The clinic gives you some guidance in telling you what's needed, but the research and choosing what you want and can pay for and how and when—that's all up to you.

Thankfully, I read contracts for a living. So, I scoured the heck out of everything. I did miss some extra costs, but it's okay. It's more frustrating than anything since you're in it now, and you're not abandoning what you set out to do—building your family. So, you pay, smile, and pray that everything will work out. You can't think of any other alternative.

At this point, we were just waiting for the sperm. My blood work and thyroid levels were great. They had to test my uterine lining and make sure there were no blockages in my fallopian tubes because I would have a harder time getting pregnant if an egg couldn't travel through one of my tubes. I could still do it if the other one was open, but it would cut my chances in half—and that's if my tubes traded off moving eggs. If they encountered a blockage, hopefully, it could be fixed. But that might be the end of the road for some people—if you have severe endometriosis, for example. It was reassuring to hear that I didn't have any issues and could proceed without intervention.

My doctor is the type who likes to do things as naturally as possible and only steps in when there is a need for it. He gave me the green light to proceed, be successful, and have a baby, and the only hormone he put me on was estrogen—to build up my uterine lining. You need your lining to be a certain thickness for the embryo to implant and become a successful pregnancy.

After month three and no success with IUI, he put me on Clomid to help me produce more eggs. Clomid also increases your chances for multiples (twins, triplets, and quadruplets). I was so excited to do this and even wondered if we would have enough time where I could do it again. *How ideal would that be?*

Then, month four went by, and I was still not pregnant. It was getting so I did and didn't want to answer the phone each time the nurse called after a pregnancy test. But more than hope, my dread was growing. After she would call, I would sit there and wonder, *why is this happening when they're implanting the sperm directly in my uterus where it's supposed to go? I have the eggs. I bought the premium sperm. What is going on with this?*

We put a lot of stock into what the doctor said about it taking after roughly five to six tries. I had to remind myself of that. So, then my thoughts would turn. *This guy is brilliant. He knows what he's talking about. Just wait for it. Five or six. Next month or the month after.*

You can understand how insane I was going. After that rallying self-talk, I would recall the rate of success—a super low 12% per try once a month—and I'm sure the hormones weren't helping.

It was like riding all the roller coasters at the park all day, every day, for months on end.

Even though Dina and I both had those faith-rattling moments, we had to be optimistic and rely on our belief that it would happen. We had to think about what our doctor had told us. And we had to allow ourselves to grieve the possibility of what could've been. It was exhausting. I told myself if IUI didn't work, we always had IVF.

It's easier to hope when you still have options.

The process outside of the implantation was wearing. We were going in five to six times every month around 7:00 a.m. I was getting poked and prodded for blood tests that checked my levels to make sure I was still on track, and I had ultrasounds to check the follicle growth and thickness of my uterine lining. Timing is key, and you must be precise when it comes to insemination.

But we got through it and still lived our life. By this time, it was summer. We were traveling and trying to enjoy the longer days and each other. We'd only been together two and a half years and had just gotten married. So much of our time had gone into trying to create this little baby; we wanted to make sure there was time for us, too. This is the definition of being drawn and quartered by your emotions.

Our first wedding anniversary came and went, and we were still not pregnant. Then, for whatever reason, I wasn't producing any follicles of significant size, and my cycle was canceled. The measurements needed to be between 19-20-millimeters, and mine just weren't growing that month.

Dina and I decided to look at this turn of events from a different angle. Now we could get away and do something for our anniversary. We didn't need to stay local and hang near the clinic. We made the best of it because we had a couple of cycles left. I was clutching hope to my chest that it would work out. Even if six wasn't a go, there was no reason I couldn't do seven. And I didn't want to do IVF, but it was an option if we needed to go there. For the break, Dina and I took off and spent the weekend in New York City, celebrating our one-year anniversary. It was perfect!

September and October went by, and we still weren't pregnant.

In November, we geared up for our sixth IUI and decided this was it. If it didn't take, we were going to transition to IVF. Yes, we thought we would do seven, but emotions and steps change throughout the process. You're just riding highs and lows like tidal waves and inch-deep water battering a shore.

The meds were taking a toll on my body, so much so that I was ready to blow up over the bloating and fatigue. Being prepped for pregnancy is like PMS but ten times worse. I didn't feel like myself, but I did feel yucky, defeated, and drained.

When Dina and I called and spoke to the doctor about moving to IVF, he told us, "Why don't you both come into the office? Let's discuss it in person."

At our appointment, our doctor did not want to give up on IUI. He gave us some information on IVF but reinforced that we needed to keep the faith for this sixth try. Dina and I did decide that if this next time was a no-go, I could take some time off and normalize my body before jumping back into filling myself up with hormones and eggs. I didn't mind the idea of a reprieve. So, November would be our last IUI. We'd take December off and resume in February, two months shy of my 38th birthday.

Since this was our last attempt at IUI, during our two-week wait, we decided to head to Miami for a quick getaway from the cold weather and stressful last couple of months. I aimed to not be so rigid and cut myself a break from following all the rules; I even had a drink or two while we relaxed by the pool and on the beach. It was the least stressed I'd felt since we'd started the rounds of IUIs. I believed we were moving on to IVF.

It was the day after Thanksgiving. I was supposed to get the call from the nurse to let us know if we were pregnant or not. I'm obsessed with Christmas usually and can't wait to get the tree. Traditionally, my mom goes with us, and we all pick out and decorate it. Dina bakes five different kinds of cookies; we listen to all the holiday jazz, and it's wonderful.

That day, I remember looking out the window right before leaving to go get the tree and saying to my mom, "I'm so tired of not getting my way." My mom said, "What do you mean?" I got all teary-eyed as I wilted into the couch and said, "I just know what's going to happen. I'm going to get the call, and it's going to be (insert mocking tone) 'I'm sorry, Angelita. Unfortunately, you're not pregnant.'"

My mom said, "Please Don't think that way. I have a really good feeling." She smiled at me like she was trying to get me to smile back.

"Well, Mom," I said, with a smirk, "You've had a really good feeling the last five times, too."

This was my last and final go around before IVF, and I was feeling all the feels.

Dina joined the conversation and said softly, "Babe, I just want us to have a good day, and whatever happens, don't let it take away from our tradition. Just promise me you will try your best."

I gave her a small smile and a hug and really tried. We went and got the tree, then came home. I was still trying. But I was also calculating the minutes until the call. *Any minute now.*

A few minutes after we walked in the door, before we could even get the tree properly set up, the phone rang. My heart stopped for the sixth month in a row. Dina and my mom swiveled their heads from the phone to me and back. I prepared for the letdown again and the nurse's words I'd heard way too many times: "Unfortunately, you're not pregnant." I couldn't bring myself to pick up the receiver.

A FLICK OF HOPE

Dina answered the call and put it on speaker. "Hello?"

The nurse said, "Hi, Angelita," but her tone was different this time, like she was hiding a smile inside it. This was the same nurse who had called me every single time. My heartbeat turned from dull, dead clangs in my chest to literally singing *oh my gosh, it's a yes!*

"I have great news for you . . ." Dina handed me the phone, and I pressed my ear to it.

"No way!"

"Yes, you're pregnant."

Chills washed over my body. I cried in the kitchen. Dina and my mom froze, watching me, smiles spreading across their faces.

Then Dina was jumping up and down as I was trying to hear the nurse's instructions about making appointments and checking blood work to ensure my levels were increasing, but I couldn't understand anything in that moment. All I knew was *I am finally pregnant. It really happened.* This was our greatest holiday blessing.

Six. He was right.

CHAPTER 5

Shadows Fall

"There is no footprint so small that it cannot leave an imprint on this world."
—Unknown

It was Thanksgiving; we rolled into December with huge grins on our faces and the greatest miracle in my belly.

To top it off, it was Christmas time, my favorite time of year. Everything was still normal. The world hadn't heard of anything called Covid—not for a few months anyway. Dina and I were living up the holiday season and going to parties with family and friends. Dina made me mocktails, and we planned our trip to New York City. Every year, we go to Rockefeller Center right after the tree is lit and spend two nights over the weekend. That year was no different. We saw the Tina Turner Broadway musical and hit a last-minute iHeart Radio concert at Madison Square Garden with Taylor Swift, Lizzo, and the Jonas Brothers, celebrating a fitting tribute to this little life.

My pregnancy was going great. I didn't have many symptoms; I was a little more tired than usual. But nothing major. Since I have

MS, I'm more tired than the average bear—so maybe I was used to the fatigue that would've dropped another woman. It's hard to say.

Despite the bit of fatigue, nothing could keep me down. *So, I'll nap a little more. I'm over the moon!* The blood tests on the baby were all coming back normal, and Dina and I had no reason to think we wouldn't get through these months to hold our baby.

About the middle of January, everything changed. I came home from work one afternoon and finished doing whatever I needed to do. Then I sat down on the couch to chill for a minute when I felt a gush.

I knew that wasn't good. Immediately, I went from trying to relax to outright shaking and panicking. *I'm having a miscarriage. I shouldn't be getting my period.* I realize that last part probably doesn't make a lot of sense, but I was unglued and in shock. I couldn't fully comprehend what was happening. At that time, I was about 9-10 weeks pregnant, and I'd had multiple ultrasounds and all the blood work needed from the fertility clinic to graduate to see my regular OBGYN. This was supposed to be a happy ending.

I was so frozen with fear that I didn't want to get up off that couch and go into the bathroom. If I had to see it, that would mean it was real. But I had to, obviously, and I couldn't put it off. I don't know if I was crying or just walking like a block of ice toward the bathroom, maybe a little of both. One of my best friends, who is the same age as me, had miscarried a year before—she was earlier than I was, about six or seven weeks—but that was all I could think about. *Now, it's happening to me.*

What I saw was not what any pregnant woman wants to see. And I had to take a picture to document it for the doctor. Dina wasn't home. I'd been craving a roasted chicken Subway sandwich—since deli meat is off limits while preggo—and she had stepped out to get it. I will never eat Subway again.

A FLICK OF HOPE

When I called Dina, she was five minutes down the road. I knew without seeing her face that her heart had dropped when she looked at the picture. I also sent it to my best friend who'd had her miscarriage because I needed some guidance, and maybe a tiny, irrational part of my mind hoped for reassurance. I didn't get that.

After I sent her the pic, I called her to get her opinion, and she said, "You need to call the emergency line because it's after hours." It was around 7:00 p.m., and like a zombie, I replied, "Okay." She said, "I don't want to scare you. A lot of women have some bleeding in pregnancy, and it's okay." Well, she was partially right. The baby was perfectly fine.

The emergency line nurse told us, "Unless you're filling up a pad every two hours, you can wait until your next appointment with your OB at his office." That was the following week, and waiting that long was ridiculous to me.

I needed peace of mind. I wanted to be seen. I needed to know that our baby girl was okay.

At that point, I didn't know it was a girl, but I *knew*. So, Dina and I kept an eye on the bleeding for the next hour or two, and it just wouldn't stop. Even if I wasn't filling up a pad every two hours, I was still going to worry about it. That's normal. Any pregnant woman will tell you that. I insisted on being seen that night.

I went into the hospital where I had recently signed up with labor and delivery to give birth, and they did an ultrasound. The baby was fine! Dina and I were shocked, but our little tadpole was kicking around in there and loving it.

One of the OBGYN doctors in the practice we belonged to was on call. She came in, introduced herself, and explained that I had developed a subchorionic hematoma.

"Wha—" was all I could say. Then I got it together, relieved to see our baby okay and get some answers, but afraid to learn more. "I have never heard of that term."

She went on, "I don't know if you know much about it. But it's basically a pooling of blood surrounding the embryo and the uterine wall. It's not normal, but it's not uncommon."

Our heads were still spinning, and our hearts were still hoping.

"What does this mean?" *What was she going to tell us—after all this time . . . no.*

She went on, "In most cases, the body will reabsorb it. It's like a blood clot in a sense, and it's unexplainable as to why it occurs. There have been a lot of studies, and no one can explain exactly why this happens. I'm sorry, but there's nothing we can do."

You can't help me?

I was so confused.

What is she saying? We have to wait and see if the bleeding will stop on its own—if my body will absorb the hematoma? What kind of plan is that?

When we got home, after the shock had worn off some, I researched that kind of hematoma and learned they occur a little more often in IVF pregnancies—although no one knows why. In writing this book, I tried to find information on their prevalence in IUI, but nothing came up. I learned that most women who had them ended up with a successful pregnancy. Their hematomas were reabsorbed into their body. Then, I read of cases that did not end well. These hematomas increase the chance of pregnancy complications--particularly miscarriage and preterm delivery.

There was nothing the hospital could do for me, so I was advised to have an ultrasound with my regular OBGYN and do a recheck in a few days. In the meantime, my doctor told me to take it easy. I didn't have to be on bed rest, but I needed to lay low, meaning no working out, no jogging, etc. My computer work was fine, but I was restricted from doing anything too active. It was refreshing having someone force me to relax—although the reason for it was terrifying.

The bleeding continued. It was gut-wrenching to see, but when I compare that pregnancy to the next one, I still had hope. The more I learned about subchorionic hematomas, the more I was positive we would still have a baby to love and hold. That's what got me through the next two weeks.

A couple of days after my hospital visit, I had my ultrasound with my regular doctor. Dina was, again, unfailingly by my side. Before we went in, we said a prayer and held hands, trying to cover our baby girl in protection. The screen told us she looked good, and the tech agreed. "She's strong. She's healthy. She's kicking. I'm pretty sure she's waving to you guys. And she's measuring right on target. Everything looks good."

It was a moment of peace. But just a moment.

Then, another awful truth slammed into us. The ultrasound tech wasn't looking so perky. Her expression changed as she moved the wand over my belly. "There are two hematomas now."

My heart sank so low—almost out of my body and onto the floor. *There's two of these God-awful hematomas?* I couldn't say a word as Dina squeezed my hand. She was a life preserver, as the tech explained, "They're decent in size. Obviously, if they're a little smaller, they're going to reabsorb quicker. If they're larger, it will take a longer time to do so."

Then my OBGYN, who makes me think of a teddy bear, came in. He spoke softly but clearly, "Angelita, I am very sorry that you are going through this. I just want you to know that we're going to do our absolute best to help you every step of the way." He looked down for a minute, then stared me straight in the eyes. "I can't tell you what's going to happen because many of my patients with this condition have come out of it just fine with babies, and some have not."

My eyes filled with tears, and when I looked at Dina, hers were welling up, too.

My doctor continued, "But we're not going there yet. Right now, I need you to go on bed rest. I'll write you a note for work, but I do not want you to go into the office. I don't want you driving. Just the motion of moving your leg from the brake to the pedal is not good. The only way we can attempt to save this pregnancy is if you reabsorb these hematomas into your body, and we don't want them growing."

Every time I learned more and more about my condition, I wished I hadn't. We went home with the barest of hope.

Now, I had a note for work, and I hadn't even told them I was pregnant. We were so early on. Most people wait until they are at least 13 weeks—when it's considered safe.

How was I going to tell my boss? Worse yet, I didn't know if I wanted to work from home. My agenda was to do everything possible to save our baby. Naturally, I had to consider my job. It was and is stressful and demanding. I didn't think that would be good for our growing girl.

Ultimately, I put our baby ahead of my job. I just picked up the phone and had a conversation with my boss. He was empathetic and sweet, saying, "You know how we feel about you. Take all the time you need. I don't want you to worry about it, and I'm so sorry to hear this. I knew you guys were trying, and we're here for you."

His words meant the world to me and made me feel at ease. That was one worry off my plate. The next two weeks on bed rest were terrible and a total mind fuck. I'm usually a very active person, but that ground to a halt, and then there was just me and all the sensations in my body and my mind running a million miles an hour.

Bed rest means bed rest. My mom came and helped because I could not do one damn thing. Dina took off work to be with me. I was allowed to go to the bathroom and shower—but I had to limit that. My doctor made it clear, "I don't even want you to go into the kitchen to make a sandwich."

It didn't matter what I did or how still I lay; I gushed blood every single time I got up and went to the bathroom. It never stopped and was terrifying because I never knew if our girl was okay in there. I wasn't to the point where I could feel movement or kicks, so there was no way of checking that she was all right except through ultrasound.

I had four ultrasounds within those two weeks—and I was ten weeks along by then. Not only that, I had to go to my OBGYN for appointments and visits, and I had to see an MFM (maternal fetal medicine specialist) because I had a high-risk pregnancy. That had nothing to do with the bleeding. After age 35, you're considered advanced maternal age, and seeing this specialist is recommended. So, I was going to twice the number of appointments. It's nice because you get more ultrasounds and see your baby frequently, but it's a lot—especially when you're on bed rest.

At 13 weeks, everything changed again. I was still on bed rest and still bleeding, but at least our baby was on the screen.

After a few minutes, the specialist came in and shot out the sun in our world. "Angelita, you have lost almost every bit of amniotic fluid. There is suspicion of premature rupture of membranes."

CHAPTER 6

The Promise

"An angel wrote in the Book of Life my baby's date of birth, then whispered as she closed the book, 'Too beautiful for Earth.'"
—Unknown

Of course, I couldn't see the amniotic fluid mixed in with the blood. Amniotic fluid is clear. But I knew something was more wrong than usual because the night before we said goodbye to our girl, I had a really high fever and body chills. When Dina came in to check on me, I said, "I don't feel well. Something is off."

She said, "Do you want to go to the Emergency Department?"

But I didn't know what to do. *Go there and sit and be seen eight hours later? Or stay home, and what I think is nothing is really something?*

After a few seconds, I told her, "Let's just see if my fever breaks and if I feel okay."

The next day, in the ultrasound room, my doctor said, "Unfortunately, with the rate of the amniotic fluid you're losing, a loss of this pregnancy is inevitable."

They took my temperature and saw my high fever. That helped my doctor determine her next words. "My recommendation is that you terminate this pregnancy because the baby cannot live without fluid. And there's no way for you to regain it. Based on your fever, I am also concerned that you are developing an infection. With your MS, you could flare badly, and we don't know if it could be a detrimental setback for you." Her words were so soft but so sharp. Her eyes filled with tears, and there we were, all crying as we stared at this perfectly healthy baby on the screen.

I'd spent my whole pregnancy with a lump in my throat. That didn't seem right.

She *recommends that I* terminate this pregnancy. *What if I don't listen to her and the medical team and do what I want? What if I just try to hold on as hard as I can?* But those were desperate thoughts, and my heart knew it. All hope was gone.

As soon as I whispered, "Okay," she said, "I'll put in orders with your OB. He happens to be at the hospital today." Everything was very local; all the offices felt like they were next door to each other. I guessed that was a good thing.

She started walking toward the door and looked back, "I'm going to get that all taken care of, but just take some time and cry. Let it out here. The only thing I ask is when you're walking out if you can possibly try and compose yourself because other patients here are high-risk, and they're going through their own issues." I didn't take offense to that, and I kind of understood it.

Mostly, I couldn't understand anything right then. I just knew we had to go quickly.

A FLICK OF HOPE

I was sick. Our baby had no chance, and once I decided it was torture living in this reality, I wanted it done. But I never wanted to do it.

Dina and I took a couple of minutes to speed-walk through our emotions, then got it together enough to sneak through the waiting area and into the car. Once we were safely inside, we bawled openly. I said, "I'm at a loss and don't know what to do."

The last two weeks of trying to keep the baby alive had been mentally exhausting. All day long, I would talk to her, telling her I was doing everything possible to keep her safe and to hang in there, but all I could think every second of the day was, *am I gonna have this baby or not?*

I did everything the doctor told me to do. I didn't move when I lay in bed because I was fearful; I channeled my energy into reabsorbing those two things. I started meditating and journaling.

The doctor called when we were in the car. He was amazing, empathetic, and respected whatever decision we were going to make.

He said, "If you want some time, go home. Think about it. But if you want me to do the D and C procedure, I am here today and tonight. But it doesn't have to be done today. Is it emergent? Is it an emergency? Sure, especially because of your situation with the fever. But you can have a little time."

"What do you think about the whole situation, and what I should do?" I asked.

"From what I'm seeing, it's inevitable that you will lose this baby. You've lost almost all the fluid. There's no point of return from that. Whether you lose the baby tonight or in a week, the baby will not make it longer than that."

That was all Dina and I needed to hear. It became abundantly clear that I was losing her and was at risk without medical intervention.

There really was no going back.

I called my mom, and she started crying, saying, "I can't lose you. I don't want anything to happen to you. This is really hard. Pray about it. Just sit in a corner with Dina and pray. Rely on your faith to help guide you guys in making the decision."

When I called a few close friends for support, they gave me similar advice. But no one can really tell you what to do in a situation like that.

When I hung up the phone, my face wet with tears that wouldn't stop, my nose all plugged up, and the biggest pit in my gut, Dina said, "Babe, I think we know what we need to do."

"Yeah, I know."

She put the car in gear, and we went home, grabbed a couple of things, and put them in a bag. But we didn't even know what to pack. There's no list for that. My mom met us at the hospital.

Everything was surreal, a blur. There was so much crying and so many emotions. We sat there for hours waiting since our doctor was on call. Finally, I was taken back and put to sleep right away.

When I woke up, I felt like I had only been out for a few minutes. I couldn't believe it. I wasn't pregnant anymore.

I was empty.

Nothing could replace that feeling. A part of me would be missing forever. My entire being was a void. To this day, I have moments when I feel like that; they even happen during times when I am the happiest. Suddenly, I'll feel an empty pit in my stomach, and I'll know why. It hovers over me and then passes.

I was very quiet on the ride home. There wasn't much to say. My mom and Dina talked in hushed voices. Mom said through her tears, "You're going to be okay. We're going to get through this."

At home, we all sat together in the living room. The only sound was the TV—but I couldn't tell you what was on. The grief was suffocating, and we were all lost in our thoughts.

In those two weeks, when it all went downhill, my brain was on overdrive. *Maybe I can keep her? Maybe I won't be able to? Maybe I'm not meant to have children.* After it all, I kept returning to the thought that haunted me the most: *Maybe I'm not meant to have children; otherwise, why is this happening to me? Why did I finally get pregnant only to lose my baby?*

The next day, Dina got up to take a shower. When she came down, she kneeled in front of me and said, "I love you, and I know how I can help you." Her words were all broken up with tears. "This entire time, I have felt so helpless watching you go through this, and then when I was in the shower, something just came over me. I got the sense that maybe I was put into your life for this reason. I love you, of course. There's no doubt about that, but there might be something more."

I just stared at her and cried. *How many tears does a person have?* I had no clue what she was getting at. But I was thinking, *why are you trying to talk to me about this right now? I just want to be quiet.*

Dina's heart was breaking as she tried so hard to make me whole again with her words. "I have this overpowering feeling that I can do this. I can carry your baby. It would be an honor."

Now, my crying turned up a notch. I became hysterical, wailing and sobbing. I couldn't believe what this woman was saying to me.

She had never wanted to carry and never had any desire to grow a child inside her body. She was 42 at this time, so hearing this was doubly shocking. No aspect of pregnancy had been appealing to her, but she loves kids. She's amazing with kids and is the greatest aunt you'll ever meet.

My mom was still there, and she ran over to hug Dina and love on her. We didn't know what was going to come out of that conversation. But even though I thought I wanted quiet to heal and process the raw, raw event we had all just lived through, it was reassuring and reconfirmed our love. We got through as Mom knew we would.

As time went on, I kept coming back to Dina's words. They brought me peace, joy, and hope. They made me feel like everything was going to be okay. Not right away, but eventually, it would. And I didn't know what would happen in our journey to make our family, but whatever it was, it would be how it was supposed to be.

After a few months, we decided to try again . . . with our new plan. Dina would carry my biological baby.

During this time, I was struck with the idea to write a book about the loss of our baby girl and our journey that had taken us to her—and would hopefully result in another child.

We named our daughter Gianna Marie. The meaning of her name is "God is gracious." I'd picked out girl names when I was young, and we loved Gianna. It was an Italian representation, and Marie is Dina's middle name. Since I'd carried my biological child, I wanted Dina to be honored—so we selected one of her names. That's also why I took her name, so she would always have her stamp on our children.

What we went through was so heartbreaking I decided that if I could save anyone even an ounce of this unreal pain, I would do it through a book.

I wanted people to feel understood on the deepest level—and never feel alone in their journey. That's the worst feeling—to be surrounded by so many loving and supportive people as you swim in grief all by yourself. To a degree, everyone experiences that, even when they share their experiences.

Life truly is all the emotions all at once. If you're going through anything like this—let yourself feel them. And as a wise friend once told me, "Allow yourself grace even if guilt is weighing you down about eventually being happy again." You should be, and you need to be. Finding happiness doesn't diminish your loss, and don't let your loss diminish you.

When I was buried in grief, it was so strong I could feel it change me. It was morphing my thoughts and making me into a person I couldn't recognize. That's the second letting go after a death—the release you have to force to save yourself.

CHAPTER 7

Hope

"But grief is a walk alone. Others can be there and listen. But you will walk alone down your own path, at your own pace, with your sheared-off pain, your raw wounds, your denial, anger, and bitter loss. You'll come to your own peace, hopefully, but it will be on your own, in your own time."
—Cathy Lamb, The First Day of the Rest of My Life

Time is not on your side when you are considered advanced maternal age, even if you are grieving.

The grieving continues no matter what you do. The loss finds you at work, at home, at the grocery store, and especially at night when everything is too quiet. But you learn to live with it side by side as the rest of your life goes on.

If we were going to build our family, the time was now. And at first, Dina was going to carry. She'd had all the tests done and passed with flying colors—despite multiple polyps.

When we were ready, I reached out to the fertility doctor and explained what had happened. He was absolutely heartbroken and said, "I need to see you guys in person. Why don't you come into the office?"

"That's great," I said. "We would like to see you, too."

In my heart, I knew we would move forward, but that visit was for comfort—on all sides. I honestly think he needed a hug as much as we did.

After we explained everything, we started talking about trying again. It was hard not to since we were sitting in his office.

At one point, he said, "I don't know how long it's going to take you guys to heal. Is this time-sensitive? Sure. But you have some time to work with to heal as best you can."

I was surprised that we were healing a lot quicker than I had imagined. It wasn't like it never happened, more like we didn't want to live back in that terrible day. We didn't run from it, but we wanted to run toward hope more—if that makes sense.

During that conversation, the attention was on Dina. We were still planning on her carrying. She is a little older, so we had some concerns, but she's in great shape, and I knew she could do it well. I also knew that she would go through with it. She doesn't make promises very often, but when she does, she always comes through. Her word is worth more than gold to me.

She'd told me since our loss, "We're going to have a baby. I promise you. Whether that's you carrying or me carrying or if we have to adopt, we're going to have a baby. You believe me, right?"

I told her, "I do because you are promising it."

A FLICK OF HOPE

As we sat in the doctor's office, I was stepping foot on a skateboard, ready to fly out from under me. A certain amount of mental preparation goes into walking on precarious territory. You have to be ready to be hopeful and heartbroken. There are the highest highs and the deepest fears, and then you must find the center of your emotions. It's the oddest balance, but you must also be grounded and do everything in your power to ensure your partner is okay, too. What a test to our marriage!

After we shared that we thought Dina should carry my embryo this time, the doctor told us there was a name for what we wanted to do. It's called reciprocal IVF, also known as co-IVF or co-maternity. I knew quite a bit about it from friends who have done it. It's pretty cool because it bonds both people to the baby and pregnancy. I am bonded because Caden came from my genes, but Dina would carry and form her own deep bond by carrying. Some women even carry each other's embryos at the same time. (If you want more information, check out cnyfertility.com/ivf.)

Once again, the doctor sent us home with information; he was super hopeful and excited for us. That helped. He saw no reason why Dina could not carry—despite her age. He said, "I'd be a little more concerned if you were coming in here telling me that now you wanted Dina to go through the IVF egg retrieval process to retrieve her eggs. You're younger, Angelita, and that's a better plan."

I couldn't believe we had to go through counseling again, but it was required. It was also the equivalent of the counselor stating, "Now, you do understand that this is your egg, Angelita. And that, Dina, you will be carrying using donor sperm. When your child is of age and starts asking questions, these are some of the ways we suggest you handle it." You just roll your eyes, get through it, and fork over $200. Again.

The information was a little different this time because the process was different, but once we sat in that office and went through the rigamarole, we were ready to go. I suppose we should appreciate the support that comes along with the process. After all, Shady Grove had to know what they were doing and why counseling was a requirement.

***

It was the same time frame but a year later. We met with the doctor in January, and around the end of February, we're going through the whole insurance dance again. By this time, Covid had hit, and some things had changed. We were always educating ourselves on what was new and how it would affect us. Fortunately for us, the state of Maryland mandates that insurance companies cover some IVF fees. We learned it's not a perfect flat rate, and it depends on how great your coverage is. Still, we got help and did learn that before my insurance would consider covering any IVF costs, I was required to go through at least six rounds of IUI. Check that box.

We had to check the financial box, too. Could we do this again? After revisiting our finances, it turned out we could.

Also, all the testing I had done before when I was going through IUI? Well, forget that. They had to put me through a whole different type of testing. It's so draining, but you do it for your future baby and your family. I mean, what else are you going to do? Go to the closest bar and get knocked up for free by some random guy? Ha!

This chapter should honestly be called "Covid C*ckblocked My Baby-making Plans." Because suddenly, it didn't matter what we wanted to do.

One day, I got a call from a nurse at the fertility clinic. She shattered us. "We're shutting down, and unfortunately, we have no idea when we'll be reopening." Another kick in the heart. *What the actual f!* I learned the clinic was only proceeding with their current patients going through cycles, but I hadn't even ordered my medications, and I was in the middle of getting further testing done.

Or maybe this chapter should be called "Everything Happens for a Reason" because, in our case, that's exactly how everything turned out—perfectly.

For the moment, however, Covid had stuck a wrench securely in our plans. We had no idea when we could resume. Patient me was growing impatient again.

Dina and I are not ones to curl up and die when disaster strikes. We made the best of it.

I set up a home office to work from home, and Dina still went into the center as the medical field is essential. I increased my workouts since we had more time on our hands, and the days stretched out longer. We took a lot of walks and ate healthier. We're healthy eaters, to begin with, but we went even harder. I had gained some weight from the awful meds, so this was our time to slow down and focus on feeling the best we could with each other.

Throughout our walking more and eating better, we had a mantra: *It's just a matter of time.* Since there was nothing we could do physically to change anything, mentally, we strove to get stronger. We prepared ourselves for the massive lifestyle change coming. And it was going to. Even on days when I let myself feel a touch of doubt, I remembered Dina's promise to me, and I would think it again: *I am going to be a mother.*

Two months later, the clinic reopened, and we were more than ready to resume. I now attribute that pending period to our ultimate IVF success. We were home so much and not breathing in as many toxins. We spent a lot of time outdoors and on our deck, enjoying the peace and quiet. Our stress levels were lower, and our diets were cleaner.

I also started acupuncture with a very knowledgeable and wonderful traditional Chinese acupuncturist with the warmest, most caring, grandmotherly vibe. Acupuncture can provide added benefits for fertility patients and even help increase their chances of success.

Then, I discovered that CoQ10 supplements could aid and support fertility for both men and women. Women with a higher concentration of this antioxidant in the fluid surrounding their eggs experienced better-quality embryos. That was all I needed to hear! I rushed over to the nearest Trader Joe's and bought the biggest bottle on the shelf.

It was a good break away from what was to come and gave us the reset we needed. During this time, we also toyed with me trying to carry again. Over multiple conversations, it began to feel like a natural decision. But right then, we were just talking. Nothing in our plans had changed—I just couldn't deny this new idea tapping at my brain. If you know us, you know that we were about to change lanes. But no matter what has happened since, I don't regret a single moment because it led us to Caden. Whatever we had to go through to get him, that's what we needed to do.

With all parts of our lives improving and strengthening, Dina and I prepared to play a physical part in the next pregnancy.

I had a successful egg retrieval—so successful that it was unexpected for me to get the results I did. Because of that, we have one more embryo left. It's been tested and is genetically normal. In fact, it's currently frozen at the clinic's laboratory, so that might be a future baby for us!

A FLICK OF HOPE

Dina needed an HSG (hysterosalpingography) test to ensure her fallopian tubes had no blockages that could hinder a successful transfer and pregnancy.

IVF is like a choreographed dance that you have to get down to a precise beat.

I had about 24 injections in my abdomen in eleven days to stimulate my body to produce as many follicles as safely as possible—to prepare for the IVF egg retrieval. Women release one follicle per month, but you want better chances than that. Again, it's a balance. You don't want to be hyper-stimulated by these medications, but you do want the best shot at raising the odds.

Normally, we would've attended a hands-on class to learn how to administer the injections and make sure we were comfortable before going home. But this was smack in the middle of the pandemic. So, we had to watch a video online on how to do it. As I was studying the steps, I broke out in a sweat. *How am I going to learn this? I'm not in the medical field.* Then I remembered *my wife does work in the medical field! Dina can draw up the injection, and I'll give them to myself.* I was so thankful to have this realization. It calmed me down somewhat.

More than anything, we wanted a baby, and when you want something so bad, you have to learn to do whatever it is and do it afraid if you need to. When I feel afraid about anything, I think of one of my favorite quotes by Franklin D. Roosevelt: "The only thing we have to fear is fear itself." I don't recall if I thought of this saying then, but looking back, it's perfect for how I felt.

The number of shots you give yourself varies based on the ultrasound and other test results, but we knew I would be getting anywhere from 20-30 shots in nine to eleven days. Yes, those are the accurate numbers. Thank goodness for our wonderful doctor and all his nurses. We had such a great team, and they helped us through it all, letting us know what meds to order and basing what we would do and when and how off a cycle calendar, which my insurance company shipped to us.

Under our doctor's direction, we learned what time to inject the medication and how many milligrams I would need. He also ensured his team updated us on meds when my levels and test results changed. Of course, I was also heavily involved in making sure the timing of the delivery of the meds was perfect, and I didn't have any delays. Otherwise, guess what? Yep, I ran the risk of my cycle being canceled. It's all very precise.

My eggs were taking their sweet time growing, but one of them turned into Caden, so I'll let it slide. I just told myself they needed extra days to mature properly.

In the meantime, the doctor was advising Dina on getting one of her polyps removed. She had a few, but he felt one might be a problem when they did her transfer due to its location. Polyps can hinder the embryo from attaching firmly to the uterine lining. Finding polyps is fairly common after you reach a certain age, so we weren't worried about that; we were trying to keep an eye on our wallets, though. It was another unexpected cost.

You might wonder why Dina was following through with this procedure to remove the polyp if I was considering carrying again. I honestly cannot answer that. We both knew I was getting closer to making the decision to officially carry, but Dina still went in. Maybe a Higher Power influenced us to proceed this way—and it would benefit us at another stop on our journey.

Once again, obstacles into blessings; they could remove Dina's polyp at the fertility clinic. This was where she felt most comfortable. Her recovery took about a day or two, and then she was back at it—in full swing once again with our baby-making plans.

The whole time she was going through her steps of the process, I told her, "Dina, please don't feel like you can't change your mind about carrying. I would never be upset with you and just want to support you. I am not going to be disappointed. I want you doing this genuinely and sincerely because this is something you want to do."

I was trying to protect her from what I had gone through. If she ever had to endure something like that and I hadn't spoken up and told her it was okay to change her mind, I couldn't have lived with myself.

Every time I brought it up, she always said, "I'm doing this because I want to, not because you asked me. Because you certainly did not ask me. This is just my calling. This is what my heart told me to do that day in the shower." *As her heart was breaking into a million pieces for me, for us.*

That was good enough for me in the moment, but my mind would wander back to carrying, and I would feel compelled to ask her again.

Fertility Journey Take 2 went on.

Our doctor recommended that they send out my eggs for testing, called PGT-A (Preimplantation Genetic Testing for Aneuploidy). It is not covered by insurance and can run several thousand dollars. You can read more about it a little later in the book and at this link: www.igenomix.com.

Once an embryo has made it to the blastocyst stage, the embryologist removes a few cells from it that are then sent to a genetics lab for testing. The test assesses if an embryo is genetically sound. In particular, the embryo is screened to detect all 23 chromosomes since the presence of them all reduces the risk of a failed cycle or miscarrying.

With our first loss still haunting us, we didn't want to take any chances. I had turned 38, and the chances were higher that we could implant a genetically abnormal embryo and have yet another loss at some point in the pregnancy.

Finally, we were all set for the egg retrieval, but because we were going through a pandemic, Dina couldn't be in the room with me. After all we had been through, we were a little sad to learn I had to go it alone.

I was crossing my fingers to get a few follicles out of the deal—even one miracle egg that would go all the way.

When I walked into the hospital to get the retrieval done, I could barely walk, and everything hurt. It felt like my stomach was hanging down to the ground, and I was so heavy and tired with no energy. If you ever see an overly pregnant basset hound on the side of the road, with her belly tickling blades of grass, that was me. The bloating from the meds is the worst part of the process. You blow up so much it makes you think and feel like you really are pregnant.

In the retrieval room, I lay there looking at the ceiling and praying to God, *please, let this be successful. Please let us get a significant number of eggs out of this.* The whole experience is taxing.

I got ready for retrieval and awaited the fertilization. The vial of sperm had already been shipped to the fertility clinic lab, per my instructions. So, my eggs were fertilized immediately after retrieval in the procedure room.

After the retrieval, the embryologist will watch your fertilized eggs grow until they reach the blastocyst stage, which takes five days.

Yay, we got 19!

I went home.

Then, we entered the dreadful five-day stage. Our clinic happens to watch the growth through day seven, which made us feel a little more reassured. It gave our little, possible embabies additional days to make it through the process.

The blastocyst cycle is nerve-wracking. You don't know what's going to happen or if anything will. We had to prepare ourselves that many of these precious pearls of life would die—because something was wrong with the egg and biology wouldn't let it grow past a certain point. It just can't survive in that state. That's a tough fact of life you can't avoid.

During those seven days, I would periodically get calls from the clinic with an update; our egg numbers were dropping from the original 19, which is normal, but when you hear they are dying off, reality sets in: *Our chances of having healthy embryos are diminishing*. It is incredibly challenging to remain optimistic while getting pessimistic news and trying to heal from the loss of your baby.

Again, I held onto the words of our doctor. He thought we would get six, maybe seven eggs out of the blastocyst stage—as statistically, that is the norm for my age. You also learn to expect that maybe one or none will come back genetically normal per retrieval attempt. I figured the doc was the expert, so that would be the case. I can't tell you how many times remembering his words has saved my sanity. During this time, I had also told myself if I needed to do a second retrieval to be successful, I would go through with it. At the end of the seven-day cycle, the nurse called and said, "Angelita, I have great news! We have five, and they're high-graded." I wrote down all the grades and was ecstatic to hear these results. I had a few AAs, ABs & BAs.

This was awesome! You would think we would be in the clear, but get ready for another weird fact about IVF. The grades don't matter. You can implant with a highly graded egg, and it might not work.

Still, we clung to hope. The next day, the five that made it would fly out for testing. Progress!

Before the nurse hung up, she told me, "The testing will take anywhere from 7-14 days." That was okay with me. It was what it was, after all. Sometimes, the only thing you can do is wait. She told me they wouldn't call until the test results came back. I felt great about our chances—even if one out of those five was all we could use.

During this wait, at the last minute, Dina and I decided to drive to Rehoboth Beach for a day trip. It was the Saturday before we would receive our results.

Rehoboth Beach is a 2-hour drive from our house. We wanted to celebrate the little victories in our path. So, we decided we would treat ourselves to Thrasher's fries, Grotto Pizza, and boardwalk ice cream.

Do you believe the Universe has a way of throwing you signs whether you are ready for them or not? I do, and it's up to us to pay attention and be fully aware of them.

We were flipping through XM radio and couldn't find any songs that made the drive more fun. Although there was excitement to get to the beach, we couldn't help but think about what had happened during this journey and the news we would receive in a few short days—which also felt like a lifetime.

Finally, we flipped to a channel that started playing "Three Little Birds" by Bob Marley. Have you ever listened to the lyrics? If so, how do you ever forget them?

It was a sign.

There the Universe was, sending us a billboard, but little did we know it then. All we knew was those lyrics wafting out of the radio—that we couldn't help singing to—put the biggest smiles on our faces and hope right back into our hearts. Today, we play Bob Marley songs for Caden, and he loves them all. It's meaningful.

Finally, once home again, we got the call from the doctor personally. His voice bubbled out on the other end of the phone: "I am just so ecstatic for you guys. Three out of the five are genetically normal." THREE!!!

Dreams of my cherished family were coming into view again. All because of those beautiful little eggies.

"You did a good job, Angelita," he told me when I asked him if my change in lifestyle had anything to do with our success. I think I just needed to hear that.

Sometimes, we all need to know we did a good job—especially when the stakes are so high.

CHAPTER 8

The First Transfer

"Something beautiful and full of light has appeared in the midst of the darkness and clouds."
—Unknown

Regardless of the idea of carrying again swimming around in my head, I was all set for Dina to carry our second pregnancy. We had masterfully jumped through more hoops than we ever wanted to see in our lives. Between me feeling like a pregnant seahorse with all my eggs weighing me down and Dina's polyp procedure, it was time to look forward to baby-making—my fave pastime.

Time was a healer. The days, weeks, and months went on, and my hope returned. Flukes happen. No one knows why, but they do, and maybe sometimes, we are not meant to know the reason for a long time down the road. I was finally okay with that and gearing up for a second try. Thank God for babies' beautiful spirits, their possibilities, and new beginnings. They can heal anything.

I credit moving through the pain, yet still processing it, with Dina and I holding space for each other to sit in whatever emotions we had.

Grief can get very dark. It changes the trajectory when someone is there to hold your hand and pull you up, so you don't sink down too deeply.

As Dina and I prepared for another pregnancy, I got off social media for a while and got into my own head, meditating and self-healing how I needed to. I read and spent quality time with myself. I was learning to silence my mind and breathe through the heaviness, so I could once again live in the light and really mean it, not just slap on a smile and deny my emotions. I didn't run away from any of the ugliness and sadness of our loss and thought about what Dina and our families had gone through. It wasn't just me trying to manage this loss; many people were deeply affected by it.

The more I thought about carrying, the more I was convinced I wouldn't feel like I had given it my all if I didn't. I hoped Dina wouldn't be shocked when I talked to her about it since I had constantly mentioned throughout this new round that I would be okay with her stepping back—and maybe that was why I brought it up—I wasn't done. I knew she would carry perfectly, but it also felt like if she went through with it, I would be giving in because of a weird occurrence that sometimes happens. *If it was weird, it shouldn't happen again, right? Right?*

This time, the echo in my head was my OBGYN's words, saying, "Angelita, what happened to you is unlikely to happen again. It's very rare and happens in about two percent of pregnancies."

One day, after enough dancing around the subject, I finally told Dina, "I think I want to do this again." Well, my asking her if she wanted to back out all those times didn't do a dang thing to prevent her shock. She goggled back at me with wide eyes. "Really." The wheels were turning in her head as she weighed what to say next. I know her very well, and that expression said, *Give me a minute.*

Of course, she was jolted. I was traumatized and heartbroken, crushed under the expectations of what I thought a normal pregnancy looked like—what I thought most people were lucky enough to experience. She was traumatized, too, but she didn't skip a beat when I changed directions on her—well, maybe a small one, but then she replied.

The next moment is one of the reasons I love her so much. Even though she might not have fully understood what was driving me, she was still fully supportive and said, "Absolutely. If that's what you want to do, and that's where your heart is, I know you can do this."

After talking it over with everyone in the family to see what they thought, they were on board, too. My mom said, "I get it, and I absolutely think you should. I would love to watch you carry a child. Of course, if Dina wants to carry, that's completely okay, too, and makes no difference to me. I know this is what you've wanted for as long as I can remember." I got where she was coming from. There is something special about watching your child carry your grandchild—at least, I can imagine there is.

I agreed with her. "I can't wait to feel all the feels, the carrying, the kicks, and everything that comes with it." Pregnancy has always seemed so natural and beautiful to me.

Then we sprang it on our doctor, who was more than happy to adjust the plan. He said simply, "If that's the route you guys want to take, certainly go that way. We'll support you."

Next, we started to prep my body for a possible pregnancy. It had been about six months since we'd lost Gianna, and I had a better mindset.

But I was about to learn that IVF is very different. It's a lot more involved than IUI. It is intrusive.

Since we were changing our strategy, we had to go back to square one with our insurances—luckily, we found that we had great coverage. The nurses also had to develop my new protocol concerning meds, the timeline of the meds, my blood work and levels, and the many ultrasounds I needed to help sustain a pregnancy.

I had about two months until it was go time, aka transfer time. During that period, I tried to lose a couple of pounds since I had gained so much from the egg-boosting shots. I started eating clean again, working out even more, and not drinking a lot. I was pumped to get my body detoxed and ready for pregnancy.

I dug in and took care of myself. Then my meds came in, and I started the process of having my first transfer with one of the viable embryos.

It sucked that we were doing this during Covid when you want to be with your spouse the most. You are literally creating and growing your family, and they are not allowed to be there. Often, throughout this process, it felt like we were alone despite an incredible milestone happening.

At least I could take a video of the transfer. They put the embryo in a tiny catheter and insert it right into your uterus. You can see the microscopic embryo flash on the computer screen—like the spark of life itself. It jumps through this little hoop, and after a certain period, it either implants or doesn't. Science is brilliant, isn't it?

As soon as I got in the car after the implantation, I shared the video with Dina. It was a landmark day in our family, and Dina had to wait outside. She was understandably emotional. Then you just go home. It's so climactic and anticlimactic.

Home was where the pineapple was.

An old wives' tale states that if you eat pineapple core, which contains an enzyme called bromelain, it will help with implantation. You can eat one slice for between six to eight days. (Did you know the pineapple is the icon of IVF? It's a powerful symbol for women struggling with infertility. Women go as far as wearing pineapple t-shirts or lucky pineapple socks or bracelets on their transfer days. Yes, I had them all. There's a ton of gear on Amazon you can buy. Walk into a fertility clinic, and you will see the pineapple. Maybe it's because a pineapple stands tall and looks as if it's wearing a crown.)

But seriously, our doctor said there was nothing we could do. Time would once again tell us what was to be. He told me in an effort to untangle my nerves, "I just want you to relax. Everything will be okay." I knew why he was taking the time to calm me down. My mind was climbing the walls. He must've seen the stress all over my face.

There's a two-week wait when you go through any type of fertility process. During that time, you could be pregnant but not know it since it's so early you wouldn't likely feel it. But if you took a pregnancy test too early, which they advise you not to do, it has a high chance of being positive. That's courtesy of all the baby-prep meds you are all hopped up on. In essence, you can have a false positive, and they don't want you to get your hopes up.

People have learned about empty hope the hard way, and it's devastating.

I'd been dutiful during my two weeks, eating the pineapple core—which is tough to choke down—and splurging on McDonald's fries, another wives' tale. It's an IVF pro tip that has to do with the salt aiding implantation and reducing bloating from all the meds. It's also a wonderful treat after putting your body through the wringer.

In particular, the PIO (Progesterone in Oil) you must inject hurts like hell because it's so thick. Since the hormone comes as a powder that's insoluble in water, it needs to be mixed with an oil to make it injectable. Sesame oil is most commonly used in the progesterone shot and is the standard of drug companies, but it's become hard to get. I won't tell you how long the needle is. Just know that you must inject it deep into a large muscle—usually the buttocks—while avoiding large blood vessels in the area. And you have to do this for up to ten weeks of pregnancy. Luckily, my protocol was once a day, but I have known some women who had to do this twice a day. God bless them!

You start the injection approximately five days before your transfer. Once the implant takes hold, your body will naturally start producing progesterone. Still, you must continue the injections as a form of supplementation for up to ten weeks. Progesterone supports the lining and helps the embryo implant.

Dina and I practiced doing these injections on an orange, of all things. She even drew a little face on it with a marker to lighten the mood. I alternated butt cheeks each night, and Dina would draw up the injection. Then, I would bend over, and we were done. We had a great system down involving heat and a lot of butt massaging—so good that I barely felt sore even after ten weeks. If you're going through this, ask me for tips; I have you covered.

With what I was putting my body through, I was ready for fries right out of the air fryer. If that was my new medicine, it was a massive improvement. You may know that Progesterone causes breast tenderness, headaches, weight gain, acne, nausea, and everything that mimics pregnancy symptoms. Can you see why I dreamed about those fries now?

This time, we went exactly against protocol and bought a home pregnancy test. It sat in our kitchen cabinet, where its very existence tortured me. I couldn't get it out of my mind, but Dina had a little more self-control.

A FLICK OF HOPE

I felt pregnant. Whether I was or not, my body didn't know the difference. My boobs were sore. I had period-type cramps, and I was so tired. But it could have all been a mind fuck and might've been all the estrogen and progesterone I was forcefully pumping into my body to assist in sustaining a healthy pregnancy. I really am a roller coaster aficionado.

We waited until Sunday afternoon to take the test—exactly six days after the transfer.

"Dina, what do you think?" I was practically bouncing out of my skin.

"I don't know what to say or do, either."

Life could change in one quick pee stream or stay the same. It was another level of agony—the good kind. But behind that was a darker layer. *What if this was all for nothing?*

That Sunday, we ran some errands and decided in the car, between all our running around, that we were going to test when we got home. We told ourselves, "Whatever the outcome, it's not real. It could say we're not pregnant, but that might mean we didn't give it enough time."

We still had a couple more days to go before I could have the blood work done at the fertility clinic that would tell me if I was truly pregnant. I'm sorry. I just couldn't wait that long. This entire process is nothing short of a waiting game beyond your control. This I had control of. *I'm testing!*

When we got home, we took the test out of the cupboard; I went and did my thing and left it in the bathroom. Dina and I laughed and cried and held each other in anticipation of what we were about to see.

I said, "I can't believe we're doing this because we said we weren't gonna test . . . ."

Dina finished my thought, "But we're doing this."

Then we laughed and cried some more as we trembled and waited for the results.

When the timer went off, I looked at her, my eyes huge in my head. "Go get it."

"No, you go get it."

We decided to both go get it. On that short walk to the bathroom, my heart fluttered around so many emotions.

Finally, I worked up enough courage to grab the stick. I couldn't believe what I was reading and blinked a few times. "It's positive!" I yelled, shaking, as she stood right there beaming her head off.

"How can I be pregnant?" It was another shocking moment. My mouth ran away before my mind could catch up. Of course, I know how. *It really worked. Again? My first attempt at a transfer?*

This is no faint line. It is bright. It is bold. I am pregnant. And it's early.

Then came the hard part, trying not to get my hopes up. This is why they tell you not to test. But I knew. *The line is BOLD*, I screamed silently. We decided to call our moms.

When I told my mom, she said, "I knew it. I just had a feeling." She started crying, and that got us going all over again.

But I had to pour some cold water on the moment.

After we hung up with our moms, I turned to Dina and asked, "What are we doing? We can't get this excited and hopeful."

A FLICK OF HOPE

My love said, "Get rid of that thought. Let's read our affirmation right now. We found this affirmation on foodsforfertility.com, printed it out, and put it on the refrigerator. We read it daily throughout our pregnancies.

Today is my day for a miracle to happen.

My body is where it needs to be to accept and carry a baby.

I am physically and emotionally strong enough to complete this IVF cycle.

I love myself.

I am proud of myself for doing everything in my power to conceive my baby.

My partner is supporting me in every way I need them to.

I have confidence in this process.

I trust my body to do what it was made to do.

Everything is exactly as it should be.

I will be a mother.[3]

And that's how we held onto hope for the second time. That beautiful moment actually sustained us through the roughest time of our lives—yet to come.

---

[3] FertileFoods. "IVF Positive Affirmations - Printable Daily Positive Affirmations for IVF Success." Foods for Fertility, March 1, 2021. https://foodsforfertility.com/ivf-positive-affirmations-printable-daily-positive-affirmations-for-ivf-success/.

CHAPTER 9

The Line is Bold

"Being pregnant means every day is another day closer to meeting the other love of my life."
—Unknown

The next couple of days were a special kind of hell. I felt pregnant, and I was determined to stay positive and excited. I tested again a couple of days later because I had to. I didn't want to. I *had* to. Anyone who has ever gone through this knows exactly what I mean. It's like another entity enters your body and controls your thoughts and body. You feel powerless, yet you have control all at the same time.

That test was positive and still bright and bold.

I had scheduled my blood work to take place before going into work. By then, driving to the clinic was dreadful. It was the same old route, but by then, I was usually sick to my stomach. What had happened had scarred me, and I felt it as I turned the car in that direction. One bad turn of events can skew your entire mindset.

Since we have gone through such loss, and in trying to literally survive, I came across this quote by author and yogi Michael Singer, who said, "The mind can be a dangerous place or a great gift." This quote resonates with me today in many areas of my life. I stop to repeat it and practice it as I need to.

That morning, I tried as hard as I could to be positive and remember our affirmation as I prepared for the appointment.

I pulled up to the clinic a few minutes early and parked. I'd scheduled my appointments out weeks in advance to ensure I always got the first appointment in the morning. That way, I didn't have to wait too long if the clinic got busy. When that happened, I got antsy because I needed to get to work. Now, I had my routine down. I parked and went to my usual side door, which was locked. *What the hell?*

I went around the building, where I ran into a girl who looked familiar. I must've looked familiar to her, too, based on the expression on her face. We started chatting after trying a couple of other doors and finding them all locked. Finally, we got into the building, and I burst out, "Do I know you? What's your name? I feel like I have seen you somewhere."

She said, "I'm Laura. Bev's wife. I don't know your name, but I've seen your pictures on social media. What are you doing here?"

My joy was boiling over again. "I'm here for my baby test to find out if I'm pregnant." I couldn't hide my little smile.

Her whole face lit up. "Shut up!"

I just laughed.

"So am I!"

"Really?"

She said, "IVF or IUI?"

"IVF!" I was on the verge of laughing, too.

"Shut up!" And then she paused a second. "Wait, so we could have the same due date?"

"Yeah . . . did you test?" *I think I know the answer.*

"I did. And I'm pregnant. Did you?"

"Yes, and I'm pregnant, too!" *I think.*

Then we were hugging each other and trying to hold back tears in the elevator.

"I guess we'll find out today," I said.

"Yes," she grinned. "But I'm here to tell you that we're pregnant." I knew she and her wife had one child—even though I had lost touch with Bev. A mutual friend who'd had twins through IUI had even told Dina and me that we should reach out to Laura and Bev as we were starting our journey, and their first child was conceived via IVF. But I always felt weird about it. I thought: *I'm not going to bother them. IVF is not an easy process.* Besides, I know myself too well. I would have bombarded them with all the questions. I hadn't talked to Bev in over 15 years, but yeah, *let me just pick your brain on something so personal.*

How ironic that we were meant to meet all along.

Laura and I got to the clinic floor and checked in. My appointment was before hers, but I still had to wait a minute. We sat there in the waiting room along with many, many other women who were there for their blood work appointments or to consult with the doctor. When I heard my name, I went in, had my test, and checked out. I walked over to say goodbye to Laura, and she said, "Good luck! We should exchange numbers?"

"Absolutely!" I gave her my digits and went on my way. She texted me as soon as she got her blood work done. I don't know how we got any work done that day because we both went back to our jobs and texted all morning long about our running into each other and the timing of everything being so cool and ironic. Then we became like besties waiting to get the news from our nurses.

Laura had a different nurse than me and was seeing a different doctor at the same clinic and location. We had our transfers on the same exact day at different times and locations but didn't know it. It's so crazy when you think about it.

Twiddling your thumbs for the nurse to call is like holding your breath for the cable guy.

They call in a certain window, and all you can do is sit there, ready to jump as soon as you hear the ring.

Normally, when the clinic called, it was between two and four o'clock. Laura and I were texting throughout the day and discussing how the clinic handles the pregnancy result calls. I mean, we were *dissecting* this thing.

She explained her theory: "Normally, the early calls are for the positive results. They are the good calls, and for whatever reason, that's what they do. The negative—not pregnant calls—are reserved for later in the afternoon."

I can't believe she picked up on that. Wow. Whether it was true or not, my anticipation grew even more.

I came so close to asking one of our nurses if they really spaced out the calls like that, but I didn't—maybe I didn't really want to know.

A FLICK OF HOPE

Dina and I had talked about what I would do when the nurse called since I would still be at the office. Of course, I over-thought the whole thing, and she, as always, maintained control.

My thoughts were scrambled. "Do I let her leave a voicemail? Maybe she can leave a voicemail, and we can listen to the message together at home?" I wish I could express enough the anxiety that goes through your mind and the little details you focus on—even when you're convinced you'll get the answer you want.

Dina was on a whole different, calmer planet. Once again, I gave thanks for her cooler, beautiful head. "You're pregnant. I don't need to hear the nurse say it. I know you are."

"Okay, so I will answer the call when it comes in."

Dina just chuckled at me.

That day, I got my call before Laura did. I was in the bathroom of all the crazy places to be—and I *knew* I was in the window, so why did I pick that time to go? I was on my way back to my office when a co-worker stopped to vent to me about her day. Then my phone went off.

I glanced down at the screen, then up at my co-worker. "I gotta go," I said.-She knew the story and everything that had happened, but I blurted out, "I was pregnant. And then the loss. And now I think I'm probably pregnant. This is the call." I pointed at the phone buzzing in my hand.

"Oh yeah," she clapped her hands. "Go get it." I dashed back to my office. Anyone catching sight of me racing down the hall probably thought, *what the hell kind of contract emergency is going on?*

Again, the way the nurse said hello gave me the news I'd anticipated. Her voice always went up an octave when she shared good news. It was one of those little signs I couldn't deny. *I'm pregnant.*

"So, you're pregnant!"

"Yes, I know!" I was so ecstatic, and then I was crying. Luckily, I remembered to shut my door.

After she gave me 15 seconds to get it together so I could remember her instructions, she said, "We need you to come back in two days to have another set of blood work done. We want to see those HCG numbers increasing and increasing significantly." I knew why she was telling me this. You can have a positive test with an ectopic pregnancy—when the implantation happens in one of the fallopian tubes. It can be deadly and is never viable, so they want to know right away." Those were the scenarios running through my head for a brief moment.

But this was it! The other thoughts went away, and I felt great about this pregnancy because my number was high, which meant the pregnancy should take. You want your number to double in two days. I wasn't worried in the least. After I called Dina, I texted Laura and found out that she was pregnant, too.

When I told Laura my number, she said it was so high. "Oh my God, maybe you're carrying twins."

Now it was my turn to say it: "Shut up!"

"No, seriously," she wouldn't be swayed. "You really might be."

The world stopped for a minute. *Twins?* "What do I do if it's twins?"

"Then it's twins. Everything happens for a reason." Two for the price of one? Let's go! I want a boy and a girl. If only it worked that way, right?

Well, IVF does actually work that way. You do have the option of finding out the gender in advance.

A FLICK OF HOPE

Even though Dina and I could figure out twins, I had been preparing myself for a single baby. I told her. "I'm only ready for one pregnancy and one fetus. That's enough. But whatever God gives us, He gives us; we'll roll with it."

When I got home that night and told Dina all about my weird day and Laura, she thought it was a friendship meant to be. I agreed.

I went back to the clinic three days later and had a blood test. My numbers were so good they could have set the curve. They were doubling just as they were supposed to, and everything looked amazing. I was starting to feel pregnant, too—and it wasn't the meds. When you know, you know.

Four weeks after the transfer, I went to the clinic for my first ultrasound and saw a tiny tadpole flicking around.

It's crazy what you can see so early on in pregnancy. You cannot only hear the fetal heartbeat, but you can see the yolk sac and gestational sac. Going through a fertility clinic gives you the luxury of having ultrasounds done much more in advance than if you were at your regular OBGYN's office. I always enjoyed that perk!

CHAPTER 10

Not Beating the Odds

"Every act of creation is first an act of destruction."
—Pablo Picasso

The feeling of this second pregnancy was almost surreal. We were excited and staying hopeful, but it was still hard to shake the fear and anxiety of the past that had crept its way into our lives. It was mere months since we had lost our baby girl.

But we talked about it like we do everything, and Dina said, "Try your best to treat this pregnancy as if it's our first. Like it's new and fresh." I knew what she was saying, and that type of energy was needed. She wasn't trying to discredit what I had been through, but we had to bring light to this new life and make it a different experience. We both agreed that we should try—that we and our baby deserved this.

My wife doesn't ask me for much, but when she does, I try to do my best to give her whatever it is. This was bigger than that. She was right. So, I tried. My first couple of weeks of pregnancy were great. It was a different pregnancy, and I had faith wholeheartedly that nothing would go wrong this time. Truly, in my gut and heart, I did not believe what had happened would happen again. I'd conceived this baby differently. We'd done testing on the embryo and had a slightly smaller chance of miscarriage.

In addition to those thoughts, my OBGYN helped me chase away any negative vibes by telling me, "What happened with your first pregnancy is unlikely to happen again in future pregnancies." *Oh, those words.*

This pregnancy was different than my first in another way, too. I had to work to get the devil trying to get in my ear off my shoulder. It was impossible to have a stainless reboot. I couldn't pretend what had happened hadn't happened. In no world was that possible, but I worked to strengthen my mind and shoo away any negative whims as fast as I could. I didn't want my baby to feel one iota of that vibration.

The world had almost returned to normal, too. The pandemic was still around, but everything was opened again, and even though we had to live with this virus, for the most part, people accepted the new normal.

I made it to twelve weeks, and we started thinking about doing a gender reveal for our close family. We felt so confident. The pregnancy was moving along, and after twelve weeks, your chances of having a successful pregnancy skyrocket. To further cement all was right and no genetic issues had been missed during the PGT-A testing, I had an NIPT (noninvasive prenatal test) done. This test is done in the beginning weeks of pregnancy, and it also determines the sex of the baby. It's very accurate.

Dina's sister found out the gender we were carrying first. She was charged with keeping the secret from us.

A FLICK OF HOPE

For the gender reveal party, we had a beautiful baby elephant cake made because I planned to do the nursery decor in yellow and gray baby elephants. It's a culture thing. I love elephants and the symbolism. They are sacred animals representing loyalty, wisdom, strength, and power and are known to bring good luck and excellent fortune. Besides, nothing is cuter than calf elephants with their big floppy ears and unusually large trunks.

We pushed the reveal date a little because we were still somewhat apprehensive about revealing too much too soon.

At 15 weeks, we planned a very intimate gender reveal with close family only. We planned to hold it on a Saturday afternoon. To prepare, Dina bought sunglasses, balloons, and hats to represent Team Boy or Team Girl.

On Friday night, I was talking with Dina and my mom and said, "I already know I'm carrying our girl." My mom said, "I feel like you are, too."

Dina raised her eyebrows. " I feel like the two of you like girls."

"No," I put my hands on my belly. "I know my body, and I am carrying a girl." Separately, I told my mom, "My first baby girl is up there, and she has sent her sister. That's who I'm carrying." I can't explain this feeling. It was almost a spiritual knowing.

I was glad not to need a boy's name because, back then, I thought boys' names were kind of boring. I didn't have a clue of one I would pick. We had already picked out this baby girl's name. It would be Addison or Madison, and her middle name would be Lynn. Eventually, our girl did become Addison Lynn.

I knew one fact about the boy's name we would choose—(even though I knew this pregnancy was not a boy). His middle name would be Joseph in honor of my brother, who I'd lost a few years back. His middle name had been Joseph, and I wanted to carry on the tradition.

After chatting up a good chunk of the night, we went to bed, and the next day, the family came over to decorate before the party. Dina left to pick up the cake, and we had a nice, mellow dinner. Everyone talked about whether they were on Team Boy or Team Girl. People were divided. It was so cute.

Then we cut the cake, and it was all pink—a little girl—just like I'd always known. I was in heaven.

Either way, I would have been overjoyed, but then I started crying and couldn't stop. It was another one of those moments where I wondered, *is this real?* We all had a great evening, and my mom stayed over. Dina got up before me the next morning as I wasn't feeling well. This pregnancy made me extremely nauseous. Some mornings were slow going.

I'm stubborn and wanted to give my body the most natural and healthiest way to carry, so I wouldn't take any medication. I suffered from weeks of vomiting until I couldn't take it anymore. I was vomiting entirely too much throughout the day, and finally, the doctor called in the medication for me. I don't know if you've ever taken these little magic pills, but they are incredible. It took about two days for them to really kick in. Then I wondered, *why didn't I do this before? I could have saved myself weeks of feeling so yucky*. I'm not sure if it will work for you if you need it, but the name of the med is Diclegis—it's a combination of vitamin B6 and doxylamine.

Besides living on pregnancy pops, ginger tea, and mints and barfing my guts out all day long, I was very close to getting diagnosed with hypertension. My blood pressure ran high at all my appointments, although this wasn't the case with my first pregnancy. I think it was due to anxiety and fear, even though I tried my damnedest to change my mentality and tell myself: *Everything's gonna be fine*. It's fascinating what your subconscious can do to you if you don't get it in check.

So, add to the anti-nausea pills, a low dosage of BP meds, and all my grand plans for the most natural pregnancy were foiled. Once we got the nausea under control, we had to play around with the BP pill dosage. They made me so sick until we got it right. I woke up with headaches every morning for a couple of weeks.

Since then, I have discovered yoga and, through it, the ability to honor what my body is telling me it wants or needs. In the past, I would've pushed the hell out of something until it fit well enough—even if it wasn't supposed to fit in the first place. I never wanted to admit that what I was doing wasn't working. Before we found the right dosage, I was stuck on those pills and trying to fight through feeling sick. When I called the doctor, and he adjusted the dose, I started to feel better.

Going back to my acupuncturist helped tremendously, too. I give partial credit to my treatments for our success in getting three perfectly healthy embryos versus what the doctors had said: "Angelita, statistically, due to your age, we can expect one genetically normal embryo or none on your first retrieval attempt. It would not be uncommon for these results."

Ironically, my acupuncturist didn't believe I was all that sick. "There's nothing wrong with your blood pressure. Stop taking that medication. You don't need it." You worry too much.

I laid there on the bed, trying to make sense of what she was saying, and argued, "The doctor told me I do."

So, I kept taking the pills and monitoring my blood pressure at home. I'd never needed to do that before, and Dina didn't and doesn't need it, so we had to buy a cuff.

I noticed a trend in my readings. At home and early in this pregnancy, my BP ran low—but still in the normal range. But at the doctor's, it measured higher. I was so fixated on these readings and trying to figure out the discrepancy that I even returned the first cuff, thinking it might have been defective. Both cuffs were good brands and not cheap. Testing at home with that second cuff proved the same results.

It was "white coat syndrome." As soon as I walked into the doctor's office, my blood pressure skyrocketed into the high 130s. Even though the doctor asked me to monitor my BP, he still had to report my BP correctly in case something happened—then he wouldn't be liable for it.

After my first experience, I didn't think I could ever walk into a baby appointment without feeling like a bundle of nerves.

But these issues were minor and manageable—so I considered myself lucky and trucked on.

The morning after the gender reveal party, since I was still super sick, I wanted to lie in bed a little longer and pray the nausea would kick rocks.

When I did get out of bed, I stood up and gushed like I had never gushed before. Blood spread all over the carpet. One second, everything was fine with no bleeding; then there was the gush. I was on such a high from the night before; then, I plummeted into total despair. *How could this be happening?*

I didn't even make it out of the bedroom before I was screaming Dina's name. She was downstairs in the kitchen, and when she heard me, she knew it wasn't good. Later, she said she knew I was bleeding because of the way I shrieked for her.

This time was so bad. When I went to the bathroom, I thought I would see a fetus because it looked like a murder scene.

A FLICK OF HOPE

Dina came up and tried to console me, but there was no consoling. I lost it. All I heard in my mind was: *This is not okay*. I called the emergency line at the doctor's office and told them what was going on, and the nurse said, "You're describing a significant amount of blood. We want you to go to the Emergency Department and check yourself in. One of our doctors will be on call, and they will meet you over there."

We rushed to the ED in a complete panic, tears falling uncontrollably. I was shaking. My stomach was mostly empty because I hadn't eaten much the night before. I was so sick and weak.

The minutes on the road getting there and meeting the technician to do the ultrasound felt like hours. Dina dropped me off at the front doors and went to park, and I was bleeding so much that between leaving our house and getting to the hospital, I had to go to the bathroom to change a double pad. There was so much blood.

It was the end. There was nothing else it could be with that much blood.

Once in the ultrasound room, Dina and I held each other's hands and prayed so hard. Our voices filled the room as we filled ourselves with prayers inside and out, joining our hearts together. We kept saying over and over again, "God, please take care of everything and allow our little girl to be okay." We were in a trance as the tech did her thing until we heard, "Your baby's okay." That's a whole other realm of relief. We went from horrified, terrified, and full of fear to her being okay. A fresh batch of tears rolled down my face.

Hearing those words was the biggest relief . . . but. And that's a full stop, full sentence (because there was always a "but" throughout this journey). These pregnancies and losses hit me so hard that I still sometimes say, "But." I am getting better thanks to my yoga teacher, who tells me, "There's no point in that way of thinking." I think the reason for this is because that word, in a way, invalidates everything that comes before it.

In my first pregnancy, I had those subchorionic hematomas, and it wasn't supposed to happen again, but we were sitting there and hearing it had. Those identical words hit like bricks falling onto my chest; I could hardly breathe.

But this time was worse. Way worse.

The development of this one hematoma happened much later in the pregnancy—my second trimester—and earlier is better because you have a stronger probability of reabsorption. With the words out of the doctor's mouth, I died inside. *I can't go through this again.*

I just wanted my doctor, who had come so highly recommended, by my side. But he was not on call that day, so another doctor had to give us the bad news.

There was also a concern about placental abruption—the placenta separating from the uterine wall. If that occurred, even more amniotic fluid could leak out. Now, it was not one thing. It was two. And I was in a worse living hell than before—and I hadn't thought that possible. I just laid there on the paper on the table and thought, *what else could go wrong? This is not gonna end well. It didn't end well the first time. Why think it's going to end well a second time?*

Being positive and telling Dina I would treat this pregnancy differently and that I would stay positive hadn't done a damn thing.

It was a big lie. It wasn't any different at all. With that shitty news, I started treating the pregnancy differently. I lived in terror for the rest of it. Our baby held on for the longest four weeks of my life until she was 19 weeks old—nearly halfway through the pregnancy.

If I thought the loss of my first baby girl was grueling, I couldn't have imagined this abyss of pain.

CHAPTER 11

I Can't Tell You How or When

"The root of suffering is attachment."
—Buddha

*W*hy was this happening to me? *I tried to do everything right. I married my dream girl. Yes, it's later in life, but I finally found her.*

Well, she found me, but it was a fairy tale relationship.

Then we got started right away building our family. We couldn't have been any more on the same page.

Regardless of my first pregnancy and the pain that lingered just below the surface, I'd tried my hardest to funnel good vibrations and health into this second pregnancy. Finding the hope to do it again was the hardest weight I'd ever lifted. Now, we were losing a child again—this one older, this one closer to her due date.

I transformed after that appointment. While I'd fought back the dark energy that had tried to fold itself around me and hold me inside after my first loss, I didn't care if it ate me alive in my second loss. Maybe that agony would be less. My faith was completely lost, too, like I was in the blackest sea.

The bleeding never stopped even as I carried on with life for the next month. Between my OBGYN and the specialist, I had three to four appointments each week. Everyone was monitoring me so closely. At any given moment, my placenta could have abrupted (detached), and I would have lost every single ounce of fluid because of the hematoma. Or I would follow the déjà vu of the first pregnancy and lose fluid constantly—until it was too late.

I was never in danger of losing my life. It was always the baby at risk. I had a very high probability of miscarrying.

My doctors suggested bedrest as much as possible. No exercising, no heavy lifting, and I had to limit time on my feet. My new schedule was: I went to work. I rested.

When you know you are buying time, you shut down. There was the tiniest sliver of a chance that if we could make it to 24 weeks, I could give birth to my fetus. The baby would have a lot of complications, and it would require all her will to survive, but there are stories of 24-weekers surviving and thriving with enough medical care. It was a waiting game.

I kept thinking, *where am I going to be when this happens? Am I going to be at work? Am I going to be at home? Is it going to be at night? Is it going to be during the day?*

I was just trying to survive and felt myself slowly detaching from Addison (yes, we had decided on her name). At first, I would talk to her, telling her we'd waited so long for her and promising her that if she made it, we would do everything in our power to give her the best life. But as time went by, I couldn't even talk to her, and I'm so embarrassed to share that. But I couldn't get closer to her. I never stopped living in fear of knowing I could lose her at any moment.

I ate to keep myself energized and to nourish Addison, but it was little to nothing as I couldn't stomach much.

While I didn't blame my doctor, I'd been given false hope—even though the odds of a hematoma occurrence were very low. You want to blame and be angry at someone. I was angry at myself and felt like my body was failing me yet again. I had to remind myself that no one can predict these things. It was our doctor's job to stay positive, and there had been no indication that this would happen again.

Dina asked if we had a chance to get to 24 weeks, and our doctor said, "We will certainly do our best," but he made it clear there could be complications for both the baby and me. He said, "Continue to rest, and don't do anything strenuous." That was it.

There was no way of knowing how long this would go on. My body was so worn out anyway from the medications and back-and-forth appointments with doctors. It wasn't supposed to be like this. We weren't supposed to be so defeated. I felt like such a failure.

All the trauma I'd gone through during my first loss resurfaced. Of course, it was probably always there, and while I'd dealt with it as best I could, we had resumed the process so soon after that first loss—a mere six months. That double whammy of emotions was crippling.

Every time I went to the bathroom, my stomach was in knots. Was there going to be blood? Was there going to be a day with no blood where everything would be okay? Where my faith could be restored? That was never the case.

Everyone kept saying to me, "You're so strong," until I didn't want to hear that word anymore.

Even though my body was failing me, I still went to work. I didn't miss one day. I just wanted to stay strong because everyone believed I was. I needed the distraction, so I woke up every morning and painted on a fake smile, pretending to the world that everything was okay. But my heart was silently breaking. Many people didn't even know I was pregnant the second time because we'd kept it under wraps to play it safe. And I wasn't back on social media yet—which was good.

When I got home from work and could finally fall asleep after crying for hours, I didn't have to think anymore. Family and friends sent flowers and gifts and were overwhelmingly supportive. But I could have been in a room full of people and still felt so alone. My most amazing wife would hold me tightly every night until I started pushing her away because I just wanted to be alone. The self-induced isolation was becoming the way I coped.

At my 19-week appointment, we learned I had less than 10% of my amniotic fluid left and was losing more every day. The loss of amniotic fluid this early on was not only dangerous for the baby but for my body. You don't want to develop an infection. At that stage of the pregnancy, the baby had no lung capacity and an extremely low heart rate. The doctors' hopes were diminishing. We knew where we were headed.

The baby was suffering; I was suffering. After that realization, I entered the same mental maze, all the while thinking: *Maybe the doctor is wrong? Maybe there will be a miracle, and I can carry?*

We were still under the touch-and-go rules of the pandemic. When it was time for the procedure, I had to go by myself to my final appointment. I went in completely numb, just making my body perform the functions of walking through the door and getting inside to where I needed to go. I was put under general anesthesia so they could remove the baby. It was November and a week and a half before Thanksgiving.

Dina asked for a picture of Addison's footprints at the hospital. She kept them, although it wasn't until a couple of months after that I could bring myself to ask Dina if I could see them. Addison's beautiful little feet are forever ingrained in my memory. I wasn't just grieving for the child we had just lost; I was grieving for the entire life we had planned for her.

After it was over and I was home, Dina and I didn't say much. We were both aching in our own ways. I was exhausted and tired of isolating and living in the bubble I'd been in for the past few months. Despite the hollow in my heart, I was still trying to be strong and pull myself out of the darkness. Somehow, I still found hope. There was a little relief in not living in fear of the unknown. Sometimes, I believed the hope I felt was present in everyone around me, and I was trying to tap into that feeling as best I could.

I feel like a terrible mother saying that, but it's real. Dina had been praying the whole time for Addison to be okay, but when we knew there was no chance for our little girl to survive, her prayers changed. She no longer prayed to save the baby. It was in God's hands, and He had the ultimate say If Addison was meant to be here with us or not. I love her for that.

I know now that our baby was not meant to be here on this Earth with us for whatever reason, and maybe we'll never know why.

But Addison has changed our lives forever. There will never be a day I don't think about her. What would she look like? *What would her personality have been like? Would she be like Caden?*

You can imagine that even though it was our favorite time of the year, we felt an overwhelming numbness. It was grueling, but we needed to be there for each other and renew our connection--which we had started losing along the way. I had isolated myself for too long. I didn't want my family, friends, and, most importantly, Dina to lose me. We wanted to try and enjoy the holidays the best we could.

Then, there was a tiny flicker of hope. The desire to be moms wasn't going away—despite our losses, we wanted this more than anything. And we both couldn't forget a picture we'd seen and revisited often.

Before we'd begun our pregnancy journey, and even before we'd moved in together, Dina had randomly texted me a sketch she had found on Pinterest of two females and a baby. The brunette was sitting on the blonde's lap, holding the baby boy. He had dark hair and was dressed in blue with a white beanie and white socks. I have since shown a few family members and friends that photo, and it's crazy how identical it looks to us. If you want to see it, visit this link: https://bit.ly/aflickofhope-image.

This Pinterest picture is a significant part of our story, so I had my cover designer recreate it to capture Dina, Caden, and myself. It is fitting, as Caden was born in December, and the picture depicts cold, snowy winter months.

As we struggled through losing Addison, Dina came up to our room one afternoon and showed me the picture again. "Do you remember this?" she asked me.

"Of course."

"What's in this picture?"

"A baby," I said around a lump in my throat.

She stared at me so lovingly then. "I can't tell you how this is going to happen or when, but we're going to have what's in this picture."

That just wrecked me. My tears overflowed at my tender wife and her giant heart. I couldn't speak but just held her and cried until I was empty. Then I went about my day until I had to stop and empty again with more tears. This was just who I was then—for a long time.

In case you're wondering, my friend Laura (who was impregnated on the same day as me) delivered a healthy baby girl named Parker on March 26th. Our due date was April 10th, but she went early with no complications. I will never forget April 10th. Laura had a great pregnancy.

CHAPTER 12

Right Under Our Noses

"Hope and fear cannot occupy the same space. Invite one to stay."
—Maya Angelou

I wanted nothing to do with carrying ever again. The pain was worse after this loss because it brought a new, relentless truth. Even though I never wanted to carry again, I still wanted to be a mom.

I told myself: *Maybe it will never happen. Maybe decades of fantasizing about it, naming my children, and seeing my face light up in dreams as I wrapped my arms around my beautiful kids have evaporated forever.*

Understandably, Dina doesn't want me ever to carry again. It was too gut-wrenching. And she is not one to say or tell me what to do, but on this, her opinion can't be any clearer. She told me that she wouldn't stop me—can you really stop anyone when it comes to this? But I can hear her words now, "I have very strong feelings toward you not trying this again."

"Right," I told her with the deepest sigh of my soul. "So, we're on the same page. I make healthy babies but can't carry very well."

"Well, let's mix it all up. We'll get a surrogate."

"Do you have money, Dina? They cost money," but then I realized, "Wait . . . you're free."

In all seriousness, she wasn't free. I had to give Dina $1,000 so she could gamble at the casino after she got pregnant. Obviously, it was a joke, but I wanted her to have it. She was doing what I couldn't, and I would've given her whatever she wanted. I gave it to her to blow on our Atlantic City trip. She had a blast playing blackjack and slots and brought back no money at all. I didn't care. I just had fun watching her while I threw back a couple of vodka sodas. I had to channel my grief into joy somehow. We had such a wonderful weekend spending quality time together.

On top of this chasm of grief, I had to fight my feelings over something else. Dina would carry, which meant I had to get over my longing to do it.

Before we agreed that she would carry, I had a lot to talk about, which involved emotions I wasn't too proud of. I wasn't sure if I would be jealous if she had a great pregnancy. How was I going to handle that? That was a real look in the mirror, and while I could understand my feelings, it didn't mean I had to like them or even be proud of them.

One thought was, *would she have a bond with our baby that I would never have?*

It was good to get in touch with those thoughts. If I hadn't, they might've run away with me. This is why Dina and I stress open communication and airing everything out—so it doesn't have any power. This was a new chance we were resuscitating. There was no room for anything but hope. It required a kind of mettle I'd never felt. And I can't speak for Dina, but I know she had to dig deep. That was it; we were going to do it, no matter what we encountered.

My head was on a loop: Why can't I carry? Why will she get to feel the kicks, and I can't? I had to come to some sort of closure with those thoughts and feelings, or I wouldn't be able to fully support her and our unborn baby.

When we decided Dina would carry, she called me at work one day and randomly said, "Do you have any curiosity whatsoever as to whether the embryos we have left are boys or girls, or one boy and a girl?"

A big smile broke out on my face. "Absolutely."

She was smiling, too. I could hear it through the phone.

I asked her, "Would you mind if I asked the nurse to send the records?"

Dina's so easy-going; naturally, she agreed.

I sent an email to our nurse, and it took a few days to come back—like waiting for the longest pregnancy test of your life—but that's when we learned we have two boys left. If Dina's pregnancy was successful, we would have a baby boy.

To reconfirm our baby's gender, we decided to do PGT-A testing. The fertility clinic uses a third party that then sends over the information to the clinic and, subsequently, the patient.

A PGT-A test is different from NIPT, although both can determine gender. You cannot have NIPT testing done unless you are actually pregnant, and it is done by a maternal blood test starting at around ten weeks of pregnancy. PGT-A testing is only done when you've had IVF and once the embryo is created. It's unique in that you don't have to be pregnant to have this test done, and it can test the cells of the embryo for gender. It's so cool what they can do!

Also, NIPT testing is normally covered by insurance, whereas PGT-A testing is not covered.

Very early in Dina's pregnancy, it was apparent she was moving through the paces the way a woman should. She had the pregnancy every woman wants with the right amount and level of symptoms that told us development was happening. She had the nausea and heartburn, but it all wrapped up as it should have, and then she felt awesome in her second trimester. I was enjoying the pregnancy right along with her.

We did have a scare about six months into the pregnancy when Dina saw blood. Then, I was thrust right back into my prior two pregnancies. My mind *reeled. What the hell is going on?*

She only bled slightly, but I was seriously traumatized, and being rational wasn't my strong suit anymore. You don't want to see bleeding in pregnancy anyway, even if it's just a little. It always gives you cause to check out what's going on and get to the bottom of it so you can control it. We were shopping at Target when she said, "I'll be right back. I need to go to the bathroom."

She didn't tell me the full story, but I later learned that she felt like something wasn't right. With my history, she didn't want to freak me out, so she silently slipped off to the ladies' room. When she came back, I didn't think anything of it. Every pregnant woman has to pee literally all the time.

Yet, I saw something was wrong. You know your person. Her expression and demeanor, everything was completely different. She told me, "I think we need to go."

Fear hit my heart. "What happened?"

A FLICK OF HOPE

"I don't want you to panic. But I had some bleeding."

I swear all the color ran out of my face. I wanted to scream and throw myself on the floor. I was sick in a hot flash. *No, this cannot be happening.* But then I had to get a grip. This was Dina, not me. *It's something else.* That thought was more of a prayer. My mind wanted to go back to the familiar tragedies.

When we got in the car, I said, "Everything's gonna be fine." I'm normally the one in panic mode, and she's the calm one, and even though she was rattled, she was still calm. Her motto should be, "We're not going to overreact until there's a reason to overreact." I followed her lead, but I also knew she needed me, and I was determined to be there for her the way she had unfailingly been there for me—even if I trembled and shook the whole time I was doing it.

I got my wits about me. "Let's call the doctor, tell them what's going on, and we'll go from there."

We left a message for the doctor, but we couldn't finish our errands because I told Dina, "The one thing I would ask is that you take it easy for the rest of the day until we hear back from him." I stated this so calmly; I was proud of myself.

This was my new yoga mentality in action. It has been profoundly life-changing, and I was so glad I had it in that moment.

We got back home, and I set Dina up on the couch immediately. I wanted her to stay put and relax. The less movement, the better. My mind raced back to what I had been told.

I felt reassured when our OBGYN called back. He said, in his very mild-mannered voice, "I don't want you guys to panic. I know everything you've been through."

Based on the amount of blood Dina had passed, he suggested we come in on Monday, which meant waiting a couple of days.

Our doctor advised, "Keep an eye on it. If it changes for the worse and becomes heavy, reach out. But don't panic. We'll do an ultrasound on Monday."

It was hard not to think about it, but we went about the rest of the weekend as calmly as possible. Dina took it easy while I handled house stuff.

We heard the greatest news when we went into the office on Monday. Dina was bleeding because of a polyp. She'd had quite a few removed—not just the one they'd advised—before they did her transfer to get her pregnant, but some they didn't bother removing because they weren't in the way and wouldn't prevent a successful implantation.

When you have polyps, and you're pregnant, you're stretching; you're growing, and this caused a 7 mm polyp located on her cervix to bleed. The doctor said removing it would be a simple procedure. "I will go in and take it out, and you'll feel a little pressure and bleed for a day or two. But you don't need to panic because you'll know it's the polyp and nothing else."

He removed it at that same appointment. When he took it out, it appeared big, even though he had said it was small. Dina couldn't bring herself to look. She was awake for the whole process, and I was reminded yet again of how strong she is. But that strength did not extend to viewing what the doctor had just excised.

As I laid eyes on it, I could see why the polyp would cause that type of bleeding. But again, I was reassured because it was nothing like what I had experienced. Dina was down for about a day, and then she went back to work.

That was our only scare. Dina rocked an amazing pregnancy and was extremely healthy. She will tell you she felt the healthiest she's ever felt in her entire life while she was pregnant. She's a healthy person, to begin with, but she stepped it up.

She didn't even start showing until about seven to eight months into it. Then, one morning, she popped. I looked at her with such joy and thought, *whoa, there really is a baby in there. Now, I believe it.*

With her minor procedure out of the way, we started planning our baby shower and found a meaningful venue. We held a large shower with about 40 people at Woodberry Kitchen. Two of our best friends and Dina's sister hosted and planned it all out. Nothing was too much for us on that day. The theme was "Fall in Love with Baby Cusatis," with blue, white, and gold pumpkin décor and lots of greenery. On the day we finally had our shower, it was gorgeous. But before we could get to showering, we had to get through a little snag.

About a week before our shower, we babysat Dina's eight-year-old and three-year-old nephews up in Pennsylvania, about an hour and 45 minutes away from us. Dina's sister and her husband were going to a wedding, and her mom couldn't watch the kids, so we offered.

Dina was really pregnant by then. We hadn't been doing much but relaxing every weekend and getting ready for the baby. We'd just been working on the nursery and putting together baby furniture in our spare time, so we were available to sit for the kids.

The plan was to spend the night, so her sister and husband didn't have to rush back to the house. We got all settled in and were all hanging out and having a great time. The boys, Dina, and I went down to the basement to watch a movie.

We'd made chocolate chip pumpkin cookies to munch on since it was close to Halloween and ordered pizza for the boys. Dina and I had a salad—okay, and a little pizza. We were getting a real feel of being parents.

Right in the middle of the movie, the eight-year-old started sneezing. We thought: *It's humid down here. He's just a little stuffy. That's October.* Then he started coughing.

He's a kid, so he wiped his nose with his hand. Then, he was touching the laptop, the remote, and the couch. His little sticky fingers were all over the place.

I looked at Dina, and she looked at me. This was when people had stopped freaking out so much about Covid. But in that moment, I said, "Covid?" "Sure is," she said jokingly. But what were we supposed to do? We'd already been exposed (if it was that) and were going to be there for a while. We gave the little guy meds since he had a headache, and he went to bed before the movie was over.

The next morning, our nephew was still feeling congested and tired, but it didn't seem out of the ordinary. We had breakfast with my sister-in-law and brother-in-law and the kids and left later that day.

On Monday, after we'd both returned to work, Dina received a call from her sister. She'd taken our nephew to urgent care, and he had tested positive for Covid. A memo from his school stated that two kids had tested positive—so that's where our nephew got it. We had to get tested. And sure enough, all the adults and our three-year-old nephew were positive.

Then, we had to make calls to all our baby shower guests. That was when you had to quarantine for ten days or whatever it was. We had to reschedule the shower, too. But most people could make the new date, so it all worked out.

I was much sicker than Dina, but I didn't care about myself and was happy to take one for the team. It was rough for two days, and then I was fine. We both lost our sense of smell and taste, which didn't stop Dina from eating, but that was short-lived and only lasted about a week and a half.

Dina and I had a good time even though we were sick. We watched movies and caught up on Netflix. We ate and drank a lot of tea. It was our last time being baby-free together, so we made the best of it.

We were actually grateful that we got Covid when we did because what if she was in the delivery room when we had Covid? I couldn't have been in there with her. We felt confident that the baby would be fine and that, hopefully, he would have some antibodies.

Thanksgiving rolled around, and it was very quiet. We didn't travel and see her parents in case baby came early. Before you knew it, we were getting ready for Christmas.

As is our tradition, the day after Thanksgiving, we got our tree and then made and decorated Christmas cookies. Her due date was December 10th; we knew it could be any day. If possible, we didn't want our boy to be born too close to Christmas.

We didn't need to worry about that. Babies come in their own time, no matter what your plans are. Her due date came and went, and no baby. I guess he needed some time to continue baking. Our biggest concern with missing the due date is that it's extremely accurate when doing IVF. They know the date of the transfer and that they're implanting a five-day-old embryo (in our case, seven days). Because of this, they don't want you to go a week past your due date.

Toward the end, the doctor monitored her closely. When they measured her cervix size, she was not dilating much. But that was okay. December 13th was approaching—her induction date. After being pregnant for so long, Dina said, "I'm ready. Let's just do this." Our OBGYN was on board and said he would try to schedule it for a day when he would be on call because "I would love more than anything to deliver your little baby. And by the way, if it were up to me, I would name the baby Charlie," he said with a smile.

Finally, he would not be Flick—but that little term of endearment had grown on me. That was the name we called Caden while he was in utero. People name their IVF embryos. It's a thing. I've heard some cute ones like Poppy and Bean. We went with Flick because when the transfer occurs, there's a flicker and a flash of light on the monitor, so the doctor can see where the embryo is inserted. The embryo itself looks like a little tadpole because it's so tiny. We knew about the flash, pop, flick thing, and I said after I witnessed it, "He's Flick." Dina said, "I love it."

Every day for ten months, it was, "Flick, Flick, Flick. "Sometimes Flicker and Flickster.

We told our friends and called him that so much that people said, " I bet you'll always call him Flick. Like, you're never going to call him Caden." Everyone was using this name Flick, and it was the cutest. I'll still sometimes say it, but I got the hang of Caden quickly. That's what happens when you fall in love with your kid.

When Dina was pregnant, that's how I thought of him—by his name, even though we had picked out two names for him. Dina really liked Gavin, but we wanted to wait until we met him and then decide. We kept both names a secret until Caden was born.

On induction day, we checked into the hospital, planning for Dina to have a vaginal delivery. Dina got her gown on, and they started the Pitocin. Thirty-six hours into it, she stalled out at seven centimeters dilated even though so many meds were pumping through her body.

Naturally, she felt like crap. She couldn't get out of bed, either, because once you have the epidural, you're stuck. She got so miserable that the doctor on call that day—who unfortunately wasn't her doctor—had to go home. Then another doctor came in, and she was wonderful. She decided to do a C-section because they couldn't keep giving her more meds, and her labor wasn't moving along as she'd hoped.

Once they got Dina in the OR, everything went so fast; it was a blur. It was super early in the morning, and we got lucky because they had a slot available. She was ready but was more scared of the surgery than of giving birth naturally.

I was with her, and everything went well. Caden arrived five days after his due date on December 15th at 8:29 a.m., a perfect 7 lbs., 10 oz., and 21 ½ inches long. When he came out, my heart swelled so much it nearly burst. People have told us many times, and I've heard this my whole life, too: "You never know love until you have a child and feel love as a mother or father." My God, when I saw him and locked eyes with him, he was crying, and he reached out to me like he was telling me he knew who I was.

The anesthesiologist took pictures for us and captured that amazing moment. The whole team was so happy for us. I'm sure they treated everyone that way. We weren't anything special, but it was nice as a same-sex couple that they didn't make us feel any different. If anything, we felt more loved.

The moment I became a mom, a massive amount of love flowed over me like I had never felt before. I never thought I could love anyone more than my wife, but this is a different love. It's much more intense. I knew immediately I would do anything for this baby. I would die for him.

I've heard that sometimes, when people bring their baby home, it can take some time to bond and let the love sink in. That's okay, of course, and it doesn't diminish the relationship in any way, but that wasn't my experience. For me, it was immediate love. He was ours. No other baby was meant to be our baby. He truly chose us. And he was finally here. When they put him in my arms, I just lost it. We were a family.

Dina was so out of it and drugged up beyond belief. She didn't show much emotion because she was so exhausted, and she hadn't even pushed. She had lost sleep for days on end. I didn't sleep much, either. It's uncomfortable at the hospital, but Caden gave me a second, third, and fourth wind. I was on the highest of highs.

Suddenly, a second later, as I cradled Caden in the operating room, all these machines started beeping, so I snapped my head toward the sound to see what was happening, and Dina was vomiting all over the table. Her blood pressure had dropped really low. My heart plummeted as I held my son close. I stared at Caden, then back at her. I didn't know where to look as I thought, *I'm losing my wife. What is going on?* My heart was racing. *Is this the way our story ends? My wife offers to carry and brings our child into this world, and then I lose her?*

It was scary to watch, but I soon learned Dina's reaction was not uncommon. The amount of medication in her body had overwhelmed her and made her super sick.

She was out of it for what felt like 10 minutes, but it was all of two minutes. Then, they cleaned her up and took her to a recovery room. They told me as I clutched onto Caden, "Everything's going to be okay. You are not going to lose her."

I was panicking, and Caden was crying. He was brand new, and the whole world was unfamiliar. He was scared and cold. I tried to send my body heat into him as Dina's heart rate normalized. She was getting more present, and finally, she could hold Caden. That was it for her. The greatest love she had ever experienced was shining in her eyes.

Dina's C-section required her to stay at least three nights. We loved all our nurses, and it felt like we were part of a giant family. A giant family that would let us sleep. All the nurses would sit with us longer than they had to—even as their pagers went off. When that happened, they would sigh and say, "I don't want to go." We would just smile. All of us felt so cared for. They showed us how to take care of a baby. Dina had some experience because of her nephews, but I didn't have any baby background besides changing a few diapers and feeding a few bottles when I was visiting other people.

Dina couldn't do a lot of moving around with the C-section. The nurses had to help her walk and get her to the bathroom. I was on baby duty, and that was fine with me! Now Dina says, "You just jumped in there and took charge. You became a mom and cared for Caden." Since we weren't breastfeeding, it was easier for me to help out. I bonded with Caden just as much as she did. Those fears and thoughts I'd had about how we would bond quickly diminished. He needed me as much as I needed him.

Dina told me, "It was awesome watching you in mommy mode. You were so inquisitive learning how to swaddle." I really was interested in everything I needed to know, and I killed it at swaddling. I would wrap Caden like a cute, tightly stuffed little burrito. It helped that everyone took such great care of us. When it was time to leave, we were truly sad.

We'd bonded with the nurses and doctors and are still Facebook friends with some of them. To this day, they will comment on our posts. They have been watching Caden grow up. A week later, we sent them a nice catered lunch because we just love them so much and wanted to thank them for their hospitality and generosity. We understand our experience could have been different, but it all came down to the care of our team. Every single person made our experience of learning to be new moms in those very early days better. We will never forget that.

It's not always that way for same-sex couples because no matter how much society progresses, we will always be different. Many doctors and healthcare workers deal with heterosexual couples, so there was always the nagging thought that they might discriminate against us. When you find out that is not the case—and better—that you are treated just like anyone else and cared for so well, you don't forget it. We never felt any sort of bias. It made our milestone experience so much more special and reduced our stress in trying to do everything perfectly for our newborn.

Our team put a song in our hearts and prepared us as best they could so we could knock this mommy thing out of the park. We felt mostly prepared. But the second we got back home, everything changed. We were mommies. On our own.

CHAPTER 13

Caden

"Sometimes the littlest things take up the most room in your heart."
—Winnie the Pooh

It was an extra magical time of the year, with Caden becoming a part of the family. We had so many emotions all day long, every day. Everything he did was amazing. *He's new. He's beautiful. He eats. He poops. He hiccups.* We ran on the adrenaline of joy for the first couple of nights. I was so confident, like, "I got this," even though we were so sleep-deprived, but then reality set in. It was a good reality but exhausting.

After about three or four days of being home, it hit me. My mind was in a fog and racing at the same time. I was not sleeping at all.

Dina and I traded off taking shifts eventually, but first, we were inseparable and did everything together. We were so excited. But obviously, we couldn't sustain that. I took the early night shift and slept during the morning. She took the opposite end of the day.

One night, about a week into it, Caden was crying, and I couldn't console him no matter what. I was going out of my mind, but I also, candidly, felt like shit.

Then the mom guilt sank in its hooks. I remembered the Sundays when we used to meal prep, lie on the couch, and watch a movie before getting ready for the work week.

Being so exhausted was hard, but of course, I would never trade those days for my time with Caden. I still wondered what it felt like to really relax. We all have these thoughts, so let yourself feel them when you do.

On those tough days, I didn't know if we were capable of doing it. *Did we really think this over?* That's the voice of exhaustion. I had heard of sleep deprivation, but if you haven't experienced it, you have no idea.

Still, we muscled through. As the days and weeks go by with your newborn, you get more and more sleep. One day, early in the morning, I caught Dina looking out the window as Caden cried. I saw the severe need for rest in her eyes. We had worked so hard to feel this way—so we felt all the things all the time, just like any other parent—along with a tinge of guilt because we wanted this so much.

Dina told me what she was thinking as she sat there, rocking and listening to Caden cry. "I wish I could go into work right now."

You're a human with basic, primal needs, so you get to think those things without beating yourself up. It's important to talk about those thoughts. Don't feel bad if you have them.

Everyone knows you wanted and want your baby, but that doesn't mean that suddenly, you stop feeling and thinking like a person.

The first two months were hard, but being in love made it easier. We were soaking up every moment of it. This is such a massive lifestyle change that no one can prepare you for. You can no longer just pick up and go. And all the changes seem to happen overnight.

When I look back now, I want those precious moments back. As much as I love his age, blooming personality, babbling, screaming, running around, and deep belly laughs, I want those days back when he was so teeny-tiny. Those days when I could smell that mesmerizing baby scent as he cooed away. When he would curl his arms and legs tightly into our chests and breathe so deeply. He was so much more dependent on us.

When he's two or three, I'll miss the days when he was eight months and a year. Motherhood truly gives new meaning to life. It's almost unexplainable. It's definitely incomparable. Dina and I are going to teach this little baby and then this little boy and this man so much. But he will teach us as much or more because he's an old soul—who's already changed our lives.

People believe in reincarnation, but that doesn't really align with my religion's covenants. Still, I know that I've met Caden before. We've crossed paths somewhere, somehow. I felt this the moment I laid eyes on him. It's undeniable in the way he studies people. Sometimes, when I squint, I swear, I catch a glimpse of this wise little old man. That's who he reminds us of. When he was tiny, I would call him my Buddha baby. Caden is so proper and dapper. His smile is so enchanting, and his eyes . . . oh, his eyes. Shakespeare said it best, "The eyes are the window to the soul." Before I was a parent and people would talk about their babies, I felt like an outsider. I didn't have the full story. Now, I get it. We totally hit the baby jackpot.

As parents, we cannot help but envision who our children will be.

At 22 months old, I see a fearless little boy with such life. Caden has such an empathetic, kind demeanor. I say this after witnessing a moment that can better illustrate what I am trying to say.

I was at my best friend's home having a playdate with Caden and her three-year-old son, Parker (a different Parker than my friend Laura's daughter). When her son started crying, Caden reached out his hand to wipe Parker's tears, and I saw his face turn sad. It was such a sweet, genuine glimpse into his heart.

Although earlier that day, he'd been a 13-month-old, jumping on top of Parker, roughhousing, wrestling his buddy, and laughing like it was all that mattered in that moment. Because it was.

Caden will make a difference in this world, and I won't push him to do it. Neither will Dina. He will do it on his own and discover how to do something really great with himself. But I wouldn't object if he became a fertility doctor.

Our journey truly taught us how to have more patience. Maybe that has a little bit to do with age, too. We are more patient beings at an older age. I look back at what I was like in my twenties, even in my mid-thirties, and I am a totally different person. Maybe it was our journey of waiting, waiting, waiting, waiting. Maybe we have a bigger, better, and greater appreciation of life because of everything we've gone through, but this time is beautiful.

It's hard, but it's so light. It's smelly, but it's aromatic—like any baby. But he's ours, so that makes it extra special.

Caden's perfect imperfections bring forth the deepest and most intimate love. He has no choice but to trust us. Being his mother is a privilege.

I'm not afraid of being a new mom or the mom I have wanted to be for so long. I am ready.

Would I have loved to have our two little girls? Yes, but I had to accept that our girls were not meant to be. Caden is himself, and the two girls all rolled into one incredible baby. He's the ideal little package. He makes me a better person. He makes me watch my temper and stop and think about how I want to react. Even if I stub my toe, I don't want to raise my voice if he's in the same room. He makes me more conscious of everything around us and what we will teach him that he will hopefully carry into his future. He makes me slow down and truly relish in the important moments. I learned to be selfless because he was born.

Dina and I went through literal hell to get to where we are today. As I sat down to write this book, I thought about how I needed to be careful with the message that everything will be okay in your journey. Sometimes, all I can think about is that we got lucky. It doesn't mean everyone will get that happy ending. I hope it happens for you, but so many people don't get to experience that. I do know how it feels not to be okay and to believe you will never find the person you used to be. I lived through some really dark days and wasn't convinced I would come out okay—but I did. So, if you need that hope stemming from my survival, take it.

Through my experience, I learned to fall in love with taking care of myself. I learned that pain turns into the most incredible experiences if we are open to seeing it. Is that why the lucky ones go through it? Life is a process of waves; you ride the highs, and you try your best to stay afloat on the lows without getting beaten up too badly.

When you get to the end of your fertility journey with everything you hoped for or not, sometimes, that's just how things work. We don't know why, and it's not a reflection of what you should have or not have in life. When I was healing from our second loss, I had to learn and realize that I would survive for me. I saw it as a position of strength.

Sometimes, we get caught up in a vision of what we thought life would look or be like. I had to learn to let go of that idealism and learn to find the goodness and joy in the story we were living. It is our story, and it is beautiful. I am damn proud of it. It is sometimes perfect, and other times it is messy.

Outside of being a mother, you're still a person with a life worth living. It can feel scary to say that and like you are releasing a dream if you don't get what you wanted—especially after you've wanted it so much. But it's even scarier not to say it and not choose you.

I don't have any regrets. I still got to experience being pregnant. I didn't get to carry to full-term; I felt everything else, but I never felt kicks, although I got very close. The doctor was surprised I hadn't felt them by the 19th week.

Toward those last appointments, he said, "You're going to feel them any day now."

I hope not, I thought, as I knew my time with my daughter was ending. Feeling her movements would have made it so much harder to say goodbye.

When Dina got pregnant, I got to experience through her what I couldn't. She wore the cute maternity clothes and felt the kicks. I never felt jealous as I worried I might've. Instead, I was flattered and blown away that she would do this for us—knowing how she had felt about carrying. She was more beautiful to me than ever.

I believe that God writes your story at birth. He knew every part of my life and how it would and will play out. He knew I wouldn't be ready for Dina at a younger age. For whatever reason, he placed me with her when we were a little older. He knew we were going to be mothers and how it would happen.

It took me some time to recover from our two losses. The year 2021 was one of self-love, self-care, and self-healing, and while I encouraged and supported Dina as she was pregnant, I spent that year getting to the healthiest place I have ever been.

A FLICK OF HOPE

I gave myself a spiritual, mental, physical, and emotional makeover.

It took me an entire year to stop calling myself a failure. After our second loss, I kept saying that word until I couldn't absorb it any deeper into my every cell. *I'm such a failure*, I would say. That was not a nice way to treat me at all.

I attribute my ability to recover to yoga and my teacher. I give such thanks for them in my life. It hit me as I was breathing deeply and learning to live with my agony: *I'm not a failure. My body works perfectly fine. It carries me daily. It maintains a very successful career. It works out. It travels. It now takes care of my family.*

Time is my teacher; through this journey, I have learned a magnitude of things. I learned to honor my body and my thoughts. I learned to give myself grace in moments when I feel myself spiraling. I learned patience.

What happened was a disease of circumstance. I'm learning to better my mind, body, and health. I'm learning what I had to endure to come out on this side. Maybe I'd be a hot mess otherwise. These tragedies might have slowed me down in a way I didn't even know I needed.

It's a beautiful transformation that I can finally see. There's no failing in any of this.

How can there be when we have Caden? Dina and I tell each other, "Alright, we're gonna catch up on *Firefly Lane or A Million Little Things*," and then we spend at least 15 minutes scrolling through the 50 pictures I took of Caden that day while talking about how perfect he is and how blessed we are. Not a day goes by that we take for granted what Caden has brought to our lives.

The appreciation we have for each other for the roles we played is monumental.

Sure, I created that baby embryo, but Dina did the hardest part—carrying him, while she thinks I did the hardest part—the retrieval. Everything else I went through only made me stronger and happier than ever. Dina reminds me that I found the motivation and strength and dug myself out of a very dark hole that some others would have fallen into and stayed inside.

Our journey gave us one more weird twist that happens when you do reciprocal IVF: I had to adopt my own son.

Now, both Dina's and my name are on Caden's birth certificate as a married couple and parents to him, but in some states, only Dina is considered his birth mother with legal rights. To protect myself, I had to legally adopt Caden as his parent.

It is called second-parent adoption and adds a layer of protection in every state and country we could travel to or live in. God forbid, we were in another country, and Caden ended up in the hospital for some reason; only Dina would be recognized as his parent. The medical staff could give me a hard time trying to advocate for him. Dina would be responsible for making all legal and medical decisions for Caden, and I would have no say.

Having this legal document ensures I have the same rights. We had to hire an attorney to file the paperwork and pay $1,800. Her name is Jennifer Fairfax, and she is an adoption attorney with Adoption & Assisted Reproductive Technology (ART) Attorneys. You can find out more information about these services on her website at jenniferfairfax.com/second-parent-adoption.

It's such BS. Caden was born from my egg, and Dina carried, grew, and protected him—*yet I have to file this paperwork*? That little obstacle was nothing compared to what we had been through. We hopped over it pretty easily.

Outside of the legalities, that paper meant nothing. We've done a complete 180 as a family. Our baby has made even the extended family so much closer. That's Caden's healing power.

My girlhood dream did come true. I pictured three babies, and that's what we were given: three pregnancies. It's just that two of our girls are in heaven.

What I had to tell myself when I truly thought I would never be a mother was *if I don't get my baby, it's not because I wasn't supposed to.*

Dina and I read a speech to each other at our baby shower. Our close friends and family knew of our journey and what it took to get there that day; the entire room teared up.

We were yet again reminded how loved we are and that we have the biggest support system you can imagine.

When we gave our little speeches in front of the crowd, it was almost like we were reading our wedding vows again. I told Dina, "I am going to thank our son every day for choosing us to be his mommies."

I've kept that promise so far. Before we put Caden to bed every night, I whisper to him, "Thank you for choosing me to be your mom."

I'm going to say it for the rest of his life.

ACKNOWLEDGMENTS

This list makes my heart swell with so much gratitude.

To my sweet wife, Dina. You are the true definition of "other half." You are my equal. You have supported me through this entire journey and beyond—through the good and bad times. Thank you for allowing me the time to go after my dream of writing this book. Thank you for always believing in me, our family, and our story. I could not be prouder of us. Your heart is so true and pure, and I am lucky to be loved by you. I love you immensely. All I can say is THANK YOU for everything–my love.

Caden Joseph, I dedicate this book to you, and I thank you. You will always be my baby boy and my little puff. As you grow older, you will face challenges in life. I want you to remember and try your best to remain true to yourself during those times. The storms will pass if you learn how to dance through them. Your laughter is my favorite sound. I hope this book helps you never forget how you came into this world and how very loved you are. I love you forever.

Evangeline Maharaj—Mom, for your unconditional love and example of what a mother is to their children. If I can be half the mother you are, I consider myself blessed. You gave me the gift of dreams and taught me the confidence to believe in them. Thank you for always supporting me, believing in me, and being my biggest fan. I love you.

In loving memory of my brother, Rolf Joseph Harris, I see you in my son every day, and that makes me smile.

To my amazing and talented publisher, Hilary L. Jastram, of Bookmark Publishing House, and her team, thank you for coaching and encouraging me along the way in writing this book. Thank you for believing in this book and going above and beyond to help bring it out into the world. It was an absolute pleasure working with you all.

To all my brilliant and most caring doctors: Shady Grove Fertility, Columbia, Maryland location—Joseph E. Osheroff, M.D., Obstetrics and Gynecology, Reproductive Endocrinology, and Infertility, and all the nurses and support team at SGF.

Francisco Rojas, M.D., OBGYN.

Howard County General Hospital, Columbia, Maryland. The doctors and nurse care team, special shout out to Debbie Leib.

Tiru Liang, CMD, L.Ac Certified and Licensed Acupuncturist.

Fairfax Cryobank (sperm bank/donor). – Fairfax, Virginia.

Jennifer Fairfax (Adoption Attorney).

Terri Sevison-Gray—You came into my life at a time when I needed you the most but didn't know it. You picked me up more times than I can count. You assured me everything was going to be okay at the end of this. You were right! You called and texted, if not every day, every other to check in. Thank you for the rare, beautiful friendship that changed my life forever. I will always be here for you.

Pamella Rostek-Kuwazaki—my childhood friend since the age of six—you taught me the true meaning of friendship. You were my biggest cheerleader. Your prayers when I lost all faith, your inspirational guidance, and your gentle push through my darkest days to keep going will never be forgotten.

Crystal Clark—my friend since the age of 15, my ride or die. Thank you for being such a great friend throughout the years and providing so much love, support, and advice during the most difficult time of my life. If it weren't for you and sending my love that message that night, this may not have been possible because I may have never met Dina. I'm so happy our boys will grow up together.

Liz Ortiz—for your strength and prayers even from afar. For allowing me to hold space without talking. For talking me into journaling and meditating throughout my lowest of times and simply just showing up for me as always.

Shelley Porter—thank you for being my mom's sounding board and friend throughout this process. She also needed someone to lean on, and I'm happy you are always there for her. Your most sincere love for all of us means the world.

Alden Caldwell, Certified Yoga Therapist—for your gentle heart and wisdom. We connected at the most perfect time. Thank you for teaching me and providing me with the tools that contributed to my healing process of mind, body, and spirit. For helping and guiding me to the healthiest and most authentic place I've been in my entire life. Yoga is forever ingrained in me.

Danielle Larned, David Cusatis, and Diane Cusatis—thank you for being Dina's rock and constant support system throughout our journey. I am honored to also call you family.

Jennifer Howard—for all your advice and support throughout the IVF process and constant encouragement that everything was going to be okay. Thanks for being such a great friend these past 20 years. Our boys are true miracles.

Laura Welch—for your support and positivity coupled with lightheartedness. I am grateful for the new friendship the journey to our babies brought us.

To the rest of our family and friends, you know who you are and how big of a role you played in this journey with us. Thank you for your continued support. We are so proud to have such a wonderful group of people who love and stand by us. We are grateful to each one of you.

To my readers—who can find a piece of themselves within these chapters. May you find the inspiration, courage, joy, and love contained within these pages. Thank you for reading and giving me the opportunity to reach out to you.

Lastly and most importantly, thank you to our donor. Without your help and selfless contribution, our son would not be here. We can never thank you enough and hope somehow, some way, you can feel the depth of our gratitude wherever you are.

ABOUT THE AUTHOR

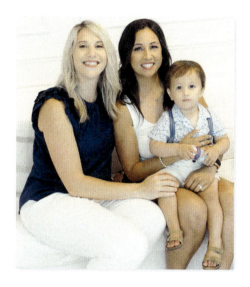

Growing up, Angelita Cusatis was an avid reader and would get excited for the summer reading list every year. She became such a voracious reader that it led to her profession as a commercial contracts manager, aka the resident bad cop.

Despite her immersion into the world of reading, she never imagined herself writing a book, much less becoming an author.

Then, she endured unforeseen events on her journey to become a mother in a same-sex relationship and knew she had to share her story. Angelita was inspired to reveal how she built her family so others struggling with loss, hope, and grief could feel her presence and know that no matter what, it is going to be okay. Her journey, although fraught with incredibly tragic turns, has forged an unbreakable bond with her wife and given her the greatest gift of all. She knows everyone's journey is different, and no matter the outcome, you must love yourself through the unpredictable and, sometimes, the unfathomable.

Angelita enjoys traveling, yoga, working out, summer mornings, reading, and doing work that leaves an impact on her community. She lives in the suburbs of Maryland with her wife, baby boy, and cute dog. You can find them traveling, cuddling, and soaking up the precious early days of their child's life as they watch him grow up too fast. This is her first book.